WALK LOSE
A HOUND A POUND

How You and Your Dog
Can Lose Weight, Stay Fit,
and Have Fun Together

PHIL ZELTZMAN, DVM, DACVS AND
REBECCA A. JOHNSON, PHD, RN, FAAN

PURDUE UNIVERSITY PRESS
West Lafayette, Indiana

Library of Congress Cataloging-in-Publication Data

Zeltzman, Phil, 1963-
  Walk a hound, lose a pound : How you and your dog can lose weight, stay fit, and have
fun together / Phil Zeltzman and Rebecca A. Johnson.
    p. cm. -- (New directions in the human-animal bond)
  Includes bibliographical references and index.
  ISBN 978-1-55753-581-8
  1. Dog walking--Health aspects. 2. Walking--Health aspects. 3. Fitness walking. 4.
Weight loss. 5. Dogs--Health. I. Johnson, Rebecca A., 1956- II.
Title.
  SF427.46.Z45 2011
  613.7'176--dc22
                            2010044573

For information, contact:
    Purdue University Press
    Stewart Center, Room 370
    504 West State Street
    West Lafayette, Indiana 47907
    www.thepress.purdue.edu

Disclaimer
The contents of this book are for personal, noncommercial, educational, and informational
purposes only. Information found in these pages and links is in no way intended to be
a substitute for professional medical or veterinary advice, diagnosis, or treatment. This
information does not constitute a recommendation or endorsement with respect to any
company, product, treatment, or procedure. The information contained herein is provided
as a public service with the understanding that Drs. Zeltzman and Johnson make no
warranties, either expressed or implied, concerning the accuracy, completeness, reliability,
or suitability of the information. Drs. Zeltzman and Johnson do not herein endorse any
commercial providers or their products.

Cover design: Mary Jane Garenda, Publications Management

Printed in the United States of America

To Alexandre and Marina, without whom I never
would have become a vet.
To Valérie, Myron, Claude, Mitch, and Bernard,
without whom I never would have become a surgeon.
—Phil Zeltzman

My work in this book is dedicated to the dogs that I
have loved and walked: Max, Jenny, Sunny, Ceilidh,
Chelsey, Ginger, Madison, and MacKenzie.
—Rebecca A. Johnson

TABLE OF CONTENTS

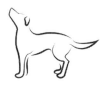

FOREWORD

"*Arf, arf, let's go for a walk. Now!*" If dogs could tell us what they want, we would be sure to hear this. In the wake of a terrible obesity epidemic in dogs and their people, we need to listen to our dogs and get busy walking them. Dogs don't like being "born retired." They have a natural inclination to get the exercise they need. If we only follow their lead, we can all be healthier and happier. This exciting new book uses research evidence to take a detailed look at the newly recognized phenomenon of dog walking as a great physical activity. For decades, people have been supersizing their hamburgers and French fries, all the while downsizing their physical activity. They have been giving their dogs too much love in the form of treats and not enough in walks and play. It's time to put a stop to these patterns that are diminishing both the quality and quantity of life for our pets and ourselves.

Walk a Hound, Lose a Pound shows how important it is for us to get up and get moving with a dog. It takes us through the process of preparing a walking program and then getting started with it. This book gives a realistic view of dog walking and provides a creative, fresh approach to it. Don't own a dog? No problem. *Walk a Hound, Lose a Pound* will tell you how you can enjoy dog walking and at the same time help a dog that needs some exercise. Shelter dogs and neighborhood pets are longing to go for a walk. They can help you get the exercise you need, while you help them become more adoptable and prepared to be a great family member. Know an older or disabled person who can't walk their dog enough? Become their dog walker and get some exercise yourself! Dogs are looking to give you unconditional love and acceptance—things that all of us need but few of us have—and they love to walk. No excuses. There are no better offers that come along that trump dog walking in terms of health benefits and general well-being. What a natural stress reliever!

In an era of economic, work, family, and internal stress, people need to be loved and to love. Walking a dog shows your love for animals, your kindness in helping neighbors and others in your community, and your belief that you are well worth taking care of. So get out there and start walking a dog, today!

DR. MARTY BECKER
"America's Veterinarian"
Veterinary Contributor to
ABC's *Good Morning America*
and *The Dr. Oz Show*
Author, columnist, and
Adjunct Professor at three
U.S. veterinary medical schools

PREFACE
Walking toward health

This book is the culmination of over three years of work formulating ideas, collecting information, drafting, and redrafting. It is meant to help people understand the significant benefits, for both people and animals, that come from regular dog walking and to get started with this enjoyable activity. It is aimed at pet lovers and may also be useful for students and practitioners in health care professions, individuals who plan and implement public health programs, and service organization staff who want to promote healthy lifestyle changes in their communities.

The collaboration between human and veterinary medicine is a natural one. The relationship between people and pets, or the human-animal bond, can be especially important in the work of health care professionals. Pets are important members of many families, and the relationships that people establish with their pets can profoundly affect their well-being, physically, mentally, and socially. As pet owners, we make commitments to our dogs; we love them and want them to be healthy. Part of this can mean that we engage in healthy behaviors that benefit both us and our dogs.

In this book we embrace One Health as a guiding principle. The concept of One Health means that people and animals experience many of the same illnesses and can benefit from many of the same solutions to live longer, healthier lives. People and animals can promote health in each other through their reciprocal bond. This strong bond contributes to the enjoyment and value of the dog-walking program we encourage for dog lovers. In this book, we do not identify the causes of weight problems in dogs and people. These causes are well known and have been described elsewhere. Instead, we discuss creative ways that people and their dogs can become fitter by exercising together and eating a healthy diet.

Dog walking is uniquely able to help promote physical and emotional health on both ends of the leash. Getting exercise while enjoying nature, giving the gift of joy to your dog or another dog in need, and interacting with other dog lovers makes dog walking a uniquely pleasurable physical activity. We believe that it can create a strong foundation for a healthier lifestyle. Scientific research proves our point, as we will show.

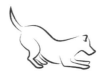

Acknowledgments

Phil Zeltzman would like to acknowledge the contribution of many pet owners, referring veterinarians, and veterinary specialists who were generous with their time and knowledge.

Rebecca A. Johnson would like to acknowledge Charlotte McKenney, Assistant Director of the University of Missouri College of Veterinary Medicine Research Center for Human-Animal Interaction, for her consistent dedication to the Walk a Hound, Lose a Pound program and study. Veterinary Medical student Annie Chih's assistance with locating resources was greatly appreciated. The author would also like to acknowledge her colleague and friend, Jackie Epping of the Centers for Disease Control and Prevention, for encouraging the program. In addition, she would like to recognize the excellent collaboration of the Central Missouri Humane Society, its Executive Directors, Patty Forister and Dr. Alan Allert, and their staff. She also recognizes the significant collaborative support of the Columbia, Missouri Parks and Recreation Department, including the enthusiasm of Karen Ramey, Erin Carrillo, and their staff members. The dedication of the Walk a Hound, Lose a Pound program and study participants helped to improve the adoptability of the more than 1000 dogs participating in the program to date. This is gratefully appreciated!

The authors would like to acknowledge Charles Watkinson, Director of Purdue University Press, for his enthusiastic support of this project. We acknowledge the dog lovers who have provided testimonials and pictures for this book. We also acknowledge the city of Lubbock, Texas, for its work with an early Walk a Hound, Lose a Pound dog-walking program and Indianapolis, Indiana for the program operated by Paula Puntenney.

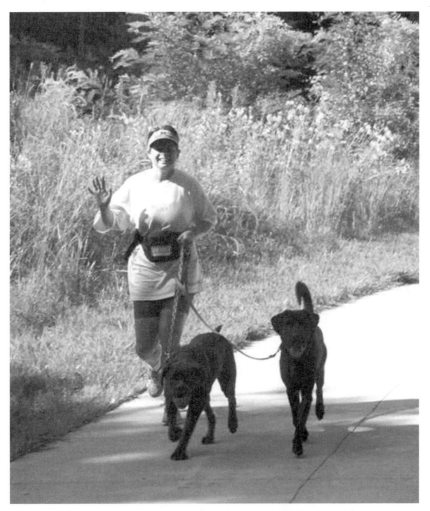

Labrador retrievers happily join in a daily jog.

1
Dog walking, the ideal activity for fitness and weight loss

You can build upon the love you share with your dog to reach a greater goal: to lose weight or stay fit. If either of you needs to lose weight or find a good way to stay in shape, walking together is an ideal solution. Because dogs and their people have similar needs for fitness and a commitment to each other, walking is a fun, fulfilling way to get exercise for both. And because walking a dog doesn't feel like exercising, it is easy to make this activity a part of your daily routine, for a lifetime of good health and companionship.

You can even walk a dog if you don't own one. Many of the concepts described in this book have been developed out of the ongoing Walk a Hound, Lose a Pound (WAHLAP) project, which takes place every Saturday from April through October in Columbia, Missouri. In this project, community residents go to the local animal shelter weekly for four weeks to walk a shelter dog for one hour. The project has been operating for four years and over 500 people have participated, helping over 1000 dogs to get their exercise, improve their leash-walking skills, and improve their socialization and chances at adoption, all the while being more physically active themselves. People who participate in the project are assessed for their physical activity levels before and after joining the program. We found that by taking a dog for a walk weekly, participants began thinking more about their own physical activity levels and became motivated to increase them. They also benefited from helping the dogs. The fun and beneficial nature of the program has been confirmed by the fact that many of the same participants return each year. They say that they like to help the dogs and that walking them is a fun activity that they can do for relaxation and interaction with their children, grandchildren, other family members or friends. The project is a simple application of the power of human-animal interaction to motivate healthy behavior in people, benefiting both ends of the leash. Programs such as WAHLAP may be helpful to increase awareness of how people can take simple steps to begin fighting the worldwide problem of obesity.[1]

The growing problem

The World Health Organization estimates that there are approximately 350 million obese people and over 1 billion overweight people in the world. Annually, about 2.5 million deaths are attributed to overweight and obesity worldwide. In the U.S., between 1998 and 2000, overweight-related illnesses cost $75 billion in medical spending.[2] Excess weight is a factor in metabolic syndrome, a collection of risk factors that increase the chance of developing heart disease, stroke, and diabetes, decreasing healthy functioning in our daily lives. More than one in five Americans has metabolic syndrome.

The rising rates of obesity in the U.S. are linked in part with limited physical activity. We need to use commonsense ways to end this dangerous trend, starting with healthy decisions about our lifestyles. As many of us know from hard experience, losing weight and then keeping it off can be difficult. Once we reach our goal weight, it is too easy to slip into our old habits. We need to find new ways to make regular physical activity a part of our lives to avoid the dangers of yo-yo dieting. Our dogs can help us do this.

Dog ownership is good for your health

Researchers have found that people who own dogs are healthier than people who don't. In one study, while the subject worked on a challenging mathematical task, the mere presence of a dog resulted in less stress and better completion of the task than when either a friend or a partner was present.[3] The physical health benefits of dog ownership partly result from powerful hormones in the blood that increase when pet owners see, touch, or smell their dogs or talk to them. The presence of animal companions helps people feel more relaxed.[4]

Dog owners are also more likely to survive after having a heart attack than those without pets.[5] Owning a dog can help to lower blood pressure, triglyceride, and cholesterol levels.[6] Scientists in Australia found that pet owners were healthier and made fewer visits to their doctor than those without pets. This saved $988 million in health care costs over one year.[7] The same trend was found in Germany, where the people who continuously owned pets were healthier and made 15% fewer doctor visits.[8]

Owning a dog also contributes to better emotional and psychological health. In fact, feeling attached to pets in general can help us feel better.[9] This has been found to be especially true for older adult pet owners and people with AIDS.[10] Owning a pet improves our morale, which is important for older adults, who are more likely to get out with a pet, stay involved with others, and participate in recreational activities rather than remain alone and inactive.[11]

Anyone who has owned dogs knows that they give us unconditional love and support, and that they are often helpful to parents in teaching children how to love, be responsible, and care for others.[12] Pets inspire us to relax and have fun and depend on us to take care of them.[13] Pet ownership can reduce anxiety, depression, and social isolation, as well as increase our physical activity.[14]

Dogs help promote conversation and other social interactions.[15] When people walk their dogs in a park, they interact more with other park users than when they walk the same route alone.[16] Dogs are conversation ice breakers. In fact, people who have a dog with them are viewed by others as more likeable than those without a dog.[17] Dog owners are more likely to do favors for one another, be more trustful of others, do volunteer work, participate in school-related activities, sports, and recreational clubs, and contribute to a sense of community than are people who do not own dogs.[18]

Dog-walking benefits for people

The U.S. Centers for Disease Control and Prevention recommend that to maintain optimal health and weight, adults need at least two hours and

30 minutes per week of moderate aerobic activity or one hour and 15 minutes per week of vigorous aerobic activity or an equivalent combination of the two.[19] Walking is an excellent way to meet this recommendation. Dog walking may be an important factor motivating physical activity, as a loving commitment to a dog involves meeting that dog's need for exercise.[20] A recent study at The George Washington University School of Public Health and Health Services examined 916 people who were either non-dog owners, dog owners who walked their dogs, or dog owners who did not walk their dogs. The study found that dog owners who walked their dogs reported fewer hours of sitting per day, a lower body mass index, lower tobacco use, fewer chronic health conditions, fewer depression symptoms, and greater social support. In addition to general fitness, then, dog walking can provide a variety of benefits for both mental and physical health.[21]

People who own dogs are more likely to meet physical activity recommendations than those who don't. In Australia, dog owners walk on average 18 minutes per week more than non-dog owners.[22] In the United Kingdom, dog owners do much more exercise than either cat owners or adults without pets.[23] In the U.S., nearly half of adults who walk dogs get at least 30 minutes of walking per day.[24] In Canada, dog owners get their recommended physical activity through dog walking; they walk an average of five hours per week, compared with three hours for non-dog owners.[25]

Dog ownership helps to foster a sense of community.[26] People who walk dogs have more contact with other people's dogs and receive even more of the benefits of human-dog contact.[27] When dog walking occurs in neighborhoods, people interact more with others and see their neighborhoods as friendlier.[28] Walking a dog may help people expand their social lives and feel more positive about where they live. Researchers in Australia found that such "social capital" is increased when people stroll through their neighborhoods with their pets. The presence of dog walkers helps to make neighborhoods seem safer, with extra eyes watching, friendlier, and more conducive to positive social interaction. People living in cul-de-sacs, which do not promote walking, have been found to have a higher body mass index. Real estate agents are finding that neighborhood walkability, in fact, has become a key factor in customers' choices. The importance of dog walking for communities is rooted in its role in the lives of individuals living in those communities. The role of dog walking through various life stages is illustrated in the testimonial below.

Owning a dog may be especially important for older adults. Cholesterol and triglyceride levels are lower in older adults who have a pet.[29] Older adults who own and walk dogs are twice as likely to meet physical activity recommendations and to have faster walking speeds than

LIFELONG DOG WALKING AND COMPANIONSHIP

At the age of 93, I reflect upon the canine companions in my life and how they partnered with me for health and happiness. First was Ted, a fox terrier. He entered my life when I was 11, saw me through college, military service, and the start of a career. No playmates of my age lived nearby in the rural Appalachian valley of my upbringing, so boyhood hikes with Ted led to a bonding and my initial sense of what that meant. Ted was my best friend.

Later Bogie, a schnauzer, came along when I was 45, and prompted a vital question: "Do I possibly have the time to walk this dog?" I had become the president of a university, with a busy wife and two children. But I knew Bogie deserved my full commitment. While all in the family took part, it was most important for me to be off each early morning and each late evening for those walks, no matter my professional and personal duties. He was an unrelentingly joyous companion and a source of relaxation.

Later followed a chapter in which our children, in maturity, shared the pleasures and benefits of having a dog in their families. At this time, Ben, an Australian shepherd, joined our household. To this day, he brings the verities in every canine soul. He shares with us his never-failing acts of love and forgiveness, compassion and gratitude, the pure joy of daily walks, and his loyalty.

—Paul, a retired university professor and lifelong dog walker non-dog owners.[30] Even for those in middle age, dog walking can help with weight loss. Overweight pet owners get more physical activity than people who don't have pets. Most of their physical activity relates to taking care of their dogs and playing with them. Research has found that dog owners are more likely, after losing weight, to keep it off for over one year when much of their activity involves their dog.[31]

Dog walking is a cheap, simple, low-impact activity that can easily be tailored to suit the needs of you and your dog. It can be done just about anywhere: in the heart of the city, in the suburbs, or in the countryside. In can be done on a sidewalk, in the park, in the woods, in the fields, around a lake, or in the mountains. Walking a dog requires few skills and is one of the cheapest ways to exercise; a leash and a good pair of shoes is all it takes to get started. You don't need any membership, special equipment, or yearly dues.

Your walking schedule should be tailored to the needs and abilities of you and your dog. You can start with short walks at the beginning, depending on your level of fitness, and progressively increase the duration. You can also increase the frequency of your walks. You may want to start with a walk every other day for a few weeks, and gradually increase that frequency to daily walks. You can walk on a flat surface in the beginning. Ideally, choose a grassy surface to reduce the stress on feet and joints—your dog's as well as yours. Your next best choice may be

THE HUMAN-ANIMAL BOND AND THE ELDERLY

When my children were young, I worked in a nursing home. The best day of the week for most of the residents was when a volunteer came with her poodle. This little dog loved everyone and always looked as though he were smiling. He could melt the heart of even the gruffest resident. Everyone always gravitated to him and wanted to pet him. I remember that there were always lots of smiles on those days.

—Christine, a Pennsylvania resident

a graveled path. Asphalt is harder on everyone's joints. Later on, as you lose weight or as you feel stronger, you can add inclines, or steps, or even running. You can also increase your walking speed as you become fitter. Ultimately, you should be able to walk briskly, which will dramatically improve your success at losing weight or staying fit.

As a low-impact activity, dog walking is suitable for overweight or obese people, people with arthritis, older adults, and people with disabilities. Be sure, however, to consult with your primary health care provider before starting any exercise program. The old "no pain, no gain" concept is no longer considered valid. There is no need to push yourself until you hurt! The more enjoyable your activity is, the more likely you will be able to make it a habit for life.

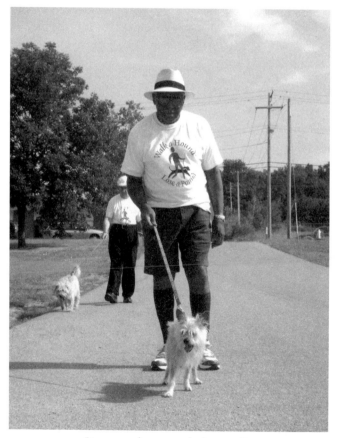

Dogs are always ready for a walk.

Dog-walking benefits for dogs

There are several scientific studies that show the multiple health benefits of walking for dogs. In one study, over 650 dog-owning households were interviewed to identify exercise, dietary, and other factors associated

TOP 10 REASONS A DOG IS THE PERFECT WALKING PARTNER

1. A dog is always ready to go.
2. A dog is a nonjudgmental partner.
3. A dog is always in a happy mood.
4. A dog will never comment on your tight, hot pink outfit.
5. A dog is never too busy and will always have time for you.
6. A dog never cancels your walk at the last minute.
7. A dog will encourage you to walk when you feel like skipping it.
8. A dog actually thinks that exercising is fun.
9. A dog never argues with you.
10. A dog won't recommend that you stop walking early to do something more urgent.

with obesity in dogs.[32] The study represented a total of 860 dogs, 25% of which were overweight. For each year of the dogs' age, the odds of obesity increased; however, for each hour of weekly exercise, the odds of obesity decreased.

Weight loss also improves comfort in dogs with hip dysplasia. A team at the University of Pennsylvania veterinary school studied 48 Lab-

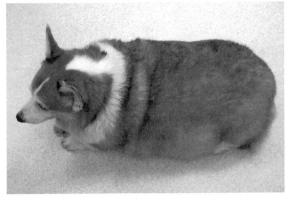

An obese corgi.

HUMAN BENEFITS OF DOG WALKING	
Weight loss	Overall well-being
Weight maintenance	Anger management
Fitness maintenance	Depression control
Immunity buildup	Meeting other people
Osteoporosis prevention	Stress and tension relief
Improvement of cardiovascular health	Insulin regulation and diabetes control
Sleep improvement	Strengthening of the human-animal bond
Anxiety reduction	
Arthritis management	

CANINE BENEFITS OF DOG WALKING	
Weight loss	Overall well-being
Weight maintenance	Anxiety reduction
Fitness maintenance	Less destructive behavior
Longer life span	Reduction in barking
Improvement of cardiovascular health	Housebreaking
Arthritis management	Improved socialization
Insulin regulation and diabetes control	Meeting other dogs
	Strengthening of the human-animal bond

rador puppies grouped in pairs of siblings.[33] Half were fed as much as they wanted, and the other half received 25% less food than their siblings. X-rays were taken over their lifetimes. At 8 years of age, heavy dogs weighed around 75 pounds, compared with 53 pounds for the light dogs, a 26% difference. The incidence of hip dysplasia increased with age: 15% at two years of age, 26% at five, 40% at eight, and 67% at the end of their lives. It is striking that hip dysplasia signs varied greatly between the two groups. One-fourth of overweight dogs were affected, but only 4% of light dogs. Even when they were eight years old, 64% of plump Labs were afflicted, versus only 14% of the thin siblings. The authors conclude that limiting a dog's food intake improves and *delays* hip arthritis.

Other researchers reached a similar conclusion. They studied 16 overweight and obese dogs with hip dysplasia. The dogs received a weight-loss diet food and walked 20 to 60 minutes every day. They lost from 9 to 27 pounds. All reached their ideal weight. Objective measurements showed that the dogs were then able to put more weight on their back legs.[34] The same researchers asked the owners of the dogs to complete questionnaires. Owners noticed an overall improvement in their pets' mobility, including less morning stiffness, an increased ability to jump into the car, and a willingness to go upstairs. Clearly, weight loss improved their quality of life.[35]

Ultimately, walking allows you to burn calories and build muscle. In dogs, weight loss is not just about quality of life. It's also about quantity of life, or lifespan. Veterinarians at the University of Pennsylvania veterinary school showed that overweight Labradors lived an average of 11 years, but their thin siblings lived an average of 13 years. This research illustrates how much truth there is to the expression "killing with kindness."[36]

Choose your partner wisely

Not every dog or every breed is an ideal walking buddy. It is important to match the type of dog to the type of activity you choose. If your goal

EXPLORING THE STREETS OF PHILADELPHIA

When I began dating my husband to be, he owned a lively little dog named Fred, a dachshund-beagle mix. To help Fred work off excess energy so that our apartment could remain destruction free, I began taking him for walks around the neighborhood. After a few walks in the early mornings, I learned how interesting a dog walk could be. Fred was a conversation catalyst. Walk him a few blocks and I would meet, and converse with, half the neighborhood. It was positively fun. Fred and I began walking regularly, exploring together the many side streets and historic alleys of Philadelphia. Together, we would try new routes and enjoy the pleasures of window shopping, discovering secret gardens, and enjoying hidden parks.

—Debra, a Pennsylvania resident

is a short, easy walk on a flat surface, almost any healthy dog should be able to join you. However, if you want to hike in the mountains for an hour every day, your Chihuahua is probably not the best choice. If your dog is very small, very large, or has major health issues, such as hip dysplasia (arthritis), heart disease, or difficulty breathing—the latter being common in flat-faced breeds—choose a different hiking partner. Athletic dogs, such as retrievers, shepherds, and sporting breeds, even if overweight, can benefit from such activities after an adequate training period.

Your dog shouldn't be too young either. Puppies have open growth plates at the ends of their bones. Growth plates are weaker areas, where cells divide to make the bones grow longer. On average, they close around one year of age, earlier in small breeds, later in large breeds. The repetitive trauma of strenuous daily walking or jogging could permanently damage a growth plate. This in turn can lead to bone deformities.

Don't have a dog? Consider other options

Obviously, you could adopt a dog. This is a serious commitment, however, and even a strong will to lose weight thanks to a dog is not a good enough reason to adopt. Other criteria should include a love for dogs, a pledge to a dog's well-being for 10 to 15 years, and the clear understanding that dog ownership is also a financial responsibility.

The benefits of dog walking can also be obtained by walking "loaner" dogs. It has been found that when older adults walked with a loaner dog, they had better heart function than after walking without a dog.[37] When overweight residents of public housing were asked to walk loaner dogs five days per week for 20 minutes, they stuck with the program, walking 72% of all possible walks. They lost an average of 14 pounds. They kept walking in the program because, as they stated, "the dogs need us to walk them."[38] The researchers also found that people who participated in a community shelter dog-walking program were motivated to increase their exercise outside of the walking program because they became aware of their need to do more exercise.[39]

Walking a loaner dog, then, can be a very healthy activity, benefiting both you and a needy dog. There are several other ways to walk a dog, even if you don't own one. You can volunteer at your local animal shelter. These dogs are desperate for exercise and companionship, and getting walks helps to make them calmer when potential adopters meet them. You can even offer to walk your neighbor's dog. If you crave the love of a canine companion but cannot own one, there are many ways for you to meet walking buddies, many of whom will benefit greatly from your attention.

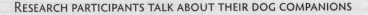

RESEARCH PARTICIPANTS TALK ABOUT THEIR DOG COMPANIONS

We had lots of fun! Every person we passed wanted to pet him!
—A satisfied dog walker

She is so responsive and remains on loose lead the majority of the time. Periodically I stop and have her come to me for snuggling . . . she makes eye contact and licks me.
—A middle-aged dog walker

It feels good being able to help my dogs get exercise, socialization with people and other dogs. I enjoy experiencing their differences, being in the company of dogs—interaction and observing them—trying to understand them.
—A dedicated dog walker

Notes

1. Johnson, R. A., & McKenney, C. (2011). Walk a hound, lose a pound: A community dog-walking program for families. In R. A. Johnson, A. M. Beck, & S. McCune (Eds.), *The health benefits of dog-walking* (ch. 6). West Lafayette, IN: Purdue University Press.

2. For global statistics on weight, see the World Health Organization web site at http://www.who.int/en. For obesity-related expenditures, see Finkelstein, E. A., Fiebelkorn, I. C., & Wang, G. (2004). State-level estimates of annual medical expenditures attributable to obesity. *Obesity Research, 12*(1), 18-24.

3. Allen, K. M., Blascovich, J., Tomaka, J., & Kelsey, R. M. (1991). Presence of human friends and pet dogs as moderators of autonomic responses to stress in women. *Journal of Personality and Social Psychology, 61*(4), 582-589.

4. Odendaal, J. S. (2000). Animal assisted therapy—magic or medicine? *Journal of Psychosomatic Research, 49*(4), 275-280.

5. Friedmann, E., & Thomas, S. A. (1995). Pet ownership, social support, and one-year survival after acute myocardial infarction in the Cardiac Arrhythmia Suppression Trial (CAST). *American Journal of Cardiology, 76*(17), 1213-1217.

6. Anderson, W. P., Reid, C. M., & Jennings, G. L. (1992). Pet ownership and risk factors for cardiovascular disease. *The Medical Journal of Australia, 157*(5), 298-301.

7. Headey, B. (1999). Health benefits and health cost savings due to pets: Preliminary estimates from an Australian national survey. *Social Indicators Research, 47*(2), 233-243.

8. Headey, B., & Grabka, M. M. (2007). Pets and human health in Germany and Australia: National longitudinal results. *Social Indictors Research, 80*(2), 297-311.

9. Garrity, T. F., Stallones, L., Marx, M. B., & Johnson, T. P. (1989). Pet ownership and attachment as supportive factors in the health of the elderly. *Anthrozoos, 3*(1), 35-44.

10. Siegel, J. M., Angulo, F. J., Detels, R., Wesch, J., & Mullen, A. (1999). AIDS diagnosis and depression in the Multicenter AIDS Cohort Study: The ameliorating impact of pet ownership. *AIDS Care, 11*(2), 157-170.

11. Lago, D., Delaney, M., Miller, M., & Grill, C. (1989). Companion animals, attitudes toward pets, and health outcomes among the elderly: A long-term follow-up. *Anthrozoos, 3*(1), 25-34.

12. Beck, A. M., & Katcher, A. H. (1996). *Between pets and people: The importance of animal companionship* (rev. ed). West Lafayette, IN: Purdue University Press; Melson, G. F. (2001). *Why the wild things are: Animals in the lives of children.* Cambridge, MA: Harvard University Press.

13. Berryman, J. C., Howells, K., & Lloyd-Evans, M. (1985). Pet owner attitudes to pets and people: A psychological study. *The Veterinary Record, 17,* 659-661.

14. Beck, A. M., & Meyers, N. M. (1996). Health enhancement and companion animal ownership. *Annual Review of Public Health, 17,* 247-257.

15. McNicholas, J., & Collis, G. M. (2000). Dogs as catalysts for social interactions: Robustness of the effect. *British Journal of Psychology, 91*(1), 61-70.

16. Messent, P. R. (1983). Social facilitation of contact with other people by pet dogs. In A. H. Katcher and A. M. Beck (Eds.), *New perspectives on our lives with companion animals* (pp. 37-46). Philadelphia, PA: University of Pennsylvania Press.

17. Rossbach, K. A. & Wilson, J. P. (1992). Does a dog's presence make a person appear more likable? Two studies. *Anthrozoos, 5*(1), 40-51.

18. Wood L., Giles-Corti, B., & Bulsara, M. (2005). The pet connection: Pets as a conduit for social capital? *Social Science & Medicine, 61*(6), 1159-1173; Wood,

L., & Christian, H. (2011). Dog walking as a catalyst for strengthening the social fabric of the community. In R. A. Johnson, A. M. Beck, & S. McCune (Eds.), *The health benefits of dog-walking*. West Lafayette, IN: Purdue University Press.

19. See the CDC's recommendations for adult physical activity: Physical activity guidelines for Americans. (2008). U.S. Department of Health and Human Services. http://www.health.gov/paguidelines/factsheetprof.aspx

20. Hoerster, K. D., Mayer, J. A., Sallis, J. F., Pizzi, N., Talley, S., Pichon, L. C., & Butler, D. A. (2010). Dog walking: Its association with physical activity guideline adherence and its correlates. *Preventive Medicine, 52*(1), 33-38.

21. Lentino, C. (2010, June). *Walk your dog to unleash better health*. Presentation at American College of Sports Medicine's 57th Annual Meeting, Baltimore, MD.

22. Bauman, A. E., Russell, S. J., Furber, S. E., & Dobson, A. J. (2001). The epidemiology of dog walking: An unmet need for human and canine health. *Medical Journal of Australia, 175*(11-12), 632-634.

23. Serpell, J. (1991). Beneficial effects of pet ownership on some aspects of human health and behaviour. *Journal of the Royal Society of Medicine, 84*(12), 717-720.

24. Ham S. A., & Epping J. (2006). Dog walking and physical activity in the United States. *Preventing Chronic Disease, 3*(2), A47.

25. Brown, S. G., & Rhodes, R. E. (2006). Relationships among dog ownership and leisure-time walking in western Canadian adults. *American Journal of Preventive Medicine, 30*(2), 131-136.

26. Wood, L., Giles-Corti, B., & Bulsara, M. (2005). The pet connection: Pets as a conduit for social capital? *Social Science & Medicine, 61*(6), 1159-1173.

27. Westgarth, C., Pinchbeck, G. L., Bradshaw, J. W. S., Dawson, S., Gaskell, R. M., & Christley, R. M. (2007). Factors associated with dog ownership and contact with dogs in a UK community. *BMC Veterinary Research, 3*(5), 1-9.

28. Wood, L., Giles-Corti, B., & Bulsara, M. (2005). The pet connection: Pets as a conduit for social capital? *Social Science & Medicine, 61*(6), 1159-1173.

29. Anderson, W. P., Reid, C. M., & Jennings, G. L. (1992). Pet ownership and risk factors for cardiovascular disease. *The Medical Journal of Australia, 157*(5), 298-301.

30. Thorpe, R. J., Simonsick, E. M., Brach, J. S., Ayonayon, H., Satterfield, S., Harris, T. B., Garcia, M., & Kritchevsky, S. B. (2006). Dog ownership, walking behavior, and maintained mobility in late life. *Journal of the American Geriatrics Society, 54*(9), 1419-1424.

31. Kushner, R. F., Blatner, D. J., Jewell, D. E., & Rudloff, K. (2006). The PPET study: People and Pets Exercising Together. *Obesity, 14*(10), 1762-1770.

32. Robertson, I. D. (2003). The association of exercise, diet and other factors with owner-perceived obesity in privately owned dogs from metropolitan Perth, WA. *Preventive Veterinary Medicine, 58*(1-2), 75-83.

33. Smith, G. K., Paster, E. R., Powers, M. Y., Lawler, D. F., Biery, D. N., Shofer, F. S., et al. (2006). Lifelong diet restriction and radiographic evidence of osteoarthritis of the hip joint in dogs. *Journal of the American Veterinary Medical Association, 229*(5), 690-693.

34. Burkholder, W. J., Taylor, L., & Hulse, D. A. (2001). Weight loss to optimal body condition increases ground reactive force in dogs with osteoarthritis [abstract]. *Proceedings,* Purina Pet Nutrition Forum, 74.

35. Burkholder, W. et al. (2002). Owner assessment points to visual improvement in signs of lameness following weight loss and increased exercise [abstract]. Purina Pet Institute.

36. Kealy, R. D., Lawler, D. F., Ballam, J. M., Mantz, S. L., Biery, D. N., Greeley, E. H., et al. (2002). Effects of diet restriction on life span and age-related changes in dogs. *Journal of the American Veterinary Medical Association, 220*(9), 1315-1320.

37. Motooka, M., Koike, H., Yokoyama, T., & Kennedy, N. L. (2006). Effect of dog walking on autonomic nervous activity in senior citizens. *Medical Journal of Australia, 184*(2), 60-63.

38. Johnson, R. A., & Meadows, R. L. (2010). Dog walking: Motivation for adherence to a walking program. *Clinical Nursing Research,19*(4), 387-402.

39. Johnson, R. A., & McKenney, C. (2011). Walk a hound, lose a pound: A community dog-walking program for families. In R. A. Johnson, A. M. Beck, & S. McCune (Eds.), *The health benefits of dog-walking* (ch. 6). West Lafayette, IN: Purdue University Press.

2

Know the health numbers for you and your dog

How does your weight compare with the average? How do you know if your dog is overweight? It is important to determine what condition you and your dog are in before starting a new regimen. This chapter examines which factors influence your health and your dog's and the ability of both of you to start a walking plan.

Below is information to help you assess what risk factors you and your pet have. The most important indicators of your health, apart from your body weight, are your waist measurement, body mass index, cholesterol profile, and blood pressure.

Health figures for you

Waist measurement

It is important to control your body weight as a risk factor. Ideal body weight varies for your gender, height, age, and ethnicity. The Resources section provides a chart of ideal body weights. An important number related to your weight is your waist measurement, because it helps you to know if your body is storing fat around your middle section. This is the most dangerous place for fat to accumulate because it surrounds important organs and can compress them or impede their function. Storing fat around your middle increases your risk of metabolic syndrome. This risk increases with a large waist. You can easily check your own waist measurement with a tape measure. Here's how:

- Remove clothing from around your middle section.
- Stand with your feet together.
- Find your lowest rib and your hip bone. Position the tape measure at the spot in the middle of these two points.
- Wrap the tape measure around your body at this spot.
- Be sure the tape measure in the back is at the same level as in the front.
- Breathe out normally.
- Bring the end of the tape measure to meet the rest of the tape measure and make it snug. This number is your waist measurement.

A measurement of over 40 inches in men and over 35 inches in women is considered a sign of overweight.

Body Mass Index (BMI)

BMI is a widely accepted way of estimating the amount of fat that you have in your body by comparing your weight to your height. BMI is not affected by age or gender but may vary for different ethnic groups. It is a way to classify your body weight as underweight, overweight, or obese. The way to calculate your BMI is to divide your weight in pounds by your height in inches, square the result, and multiply by a conversion factor of 703. The formula is written as [Weight (lb.) x 703] ÷ [height (in.)]^2.

INTERPRETING YOUR BMI

Condition	BMI
Underweight	Below 18.5
Normal	18.5 - 24.9
Overweight	25 - 29.9
Obesity (Class 1)	30 – 34.9
Obesity (Class 2)	35 – 39.9
Extreme obesity (Class 3)	Above 40

Alternatively, you can type the words "calculate my BMI" in an internet search engine. You will find websites where you can simply enter your weight and height and your BMI will be calculated automatically. One website operated by the CDC is http://www.cdc.gov/healthyweight/assessing/BMI/.

According to the World Health Organization, if your BMI is greater than or equal to 30, you are considered obese and if your BMI is 25 to 29.9, you are overweight. If you are overweight and have two or more risk factors, like high blood pressure, high cholesterol, a family history of heart disease, or smoking, or if you are a man over 45 or a woman over 55, then weight loss is highly recommended. Even a small weight loss—just 10 percent of your current weight—will help to lower your risk of developing diseases associated with obesity.[1]

Cholesterol

Cholesterol is fat that is in your blood. You need fat carried to your organs to help your body make things like the insulation on the outside of your nerves. Having fat in your blood is normal, but having too much leads to heart disease or strokes. Total cholesterol levels have become less important than the levels of each type of cholesterol. But generally, less than 200 is considered desirable, 200-239 is considered a significant risk for heart disease, and 240 and over is considered a high risk. There are two types of cholesterol, one considered good and one bad.

It can be confusing to remember which is which. One easy way to remember is that you want your HDL to be High and your LDL to be Low.

HDL, or good cholesterol

HDL stands for High-Density Lipoprotein. This cholesterol does not build up in your blood vessels, but actually helps to clear out the bad cholesterol, so higher levels are better. In the average man, HDL cholesterol levels range from 40 to 50 milligrams per deciliter (mg/dl). In the average woman, they range from 50 to 60. A HDL cholesterol of 60 or higher gives some protection against heart disease. Low HDL cholesterol (less than 40 for men, less than 50 for women) puts you at higher risk for heart disease.[2] You can increase your HDL levels with aerobic exercise.

INTERPRETING YOUR LDL CHOLESTEROL LEVELS

LDL Cholesterol Levels (mg/dl)	Rating
Less than 100	Optimal
100 to 129	Near Optimal
130 to 159	Borderline High
160 to 189	High
190 and above	Very High

LDL, or bad cholesterol

LDL stands for Low-Density Lipoprotein. The lower your LDL cholesterol, the lower your risk of heart attack and stroke. In fact, it is a better gauge of risk than total blood cholesterol. The American Heart Association uses the categories shown above to interpret LDL levels. You can decrease your LDL levels by exercising more and eating a low-fat diet rich in fruits and vegetables.[3]

Blood pressure

Blood pressure is the force that your blood makes against your arteries. It consists of two numbers. The systolic, the first number, is the pressure against your arteries when your heart beats. The diastolic, the second number, is the pressure against your arteries when your heart rests between beats. High blood pressure levels in either of these numbers mean that you are at higher risk for having a stroke. If your blood pressure is in the prehypertension range or above, your health care provider needs to evaluate whether or not you need to take medication. If your blood pressure is high to any degree, losing weight may help to bring it down.[4]

Taken together, your health numbers will help you know if your body is within a healthy range. If it is not, then you can still reduce your

INTERPRETING YOUR BLOOD PRESSURE

Blood pressure category	Systolic (mm Hg)	Diastolic (mmHg)
Normal	less than 120	less than 80
Prehypertension	120–139	80–89
High, stage 1	140–159	90-99
High, stage 2	160 or higher	100 or higher

risk of developing the devastating conditions that are related to over-weight and obesity. The first step in doing this is reviewing your num-bers. It will help if you record your health numbers on a simple form so that you can see them all in one place. There is a table included in the Resources section at the end of this book to help you do that.

Health figures for your dog

Now that you have taken an honest look at yourself, let's assess your dog. How can you tell if your pet is overweight? Some pet owners are per-fectly aware that their pet needs to lose weight. However, a fair number seem surprised when they hear from their veterinarian that their pet is overweight. Granted, it can be tricky to realize a pet has gained weight. Some breeds are so hairy—Newfoundlands, golden retrievers, collies—that it can be difficult to become aware of the problem. But it is critical for dog owners to objectively assess their pet's weight.

Your pet's activity

The cause of overweight is simple, really: it occurs when dogs eat more calories than they need. They just eat too much or they don't have enough activity to burn off the calories.[5]

Pet owners give a variety of excuses to explain why their dog is over-weight. Patty Khuly lists 10 classic excuses in her witty daily blog at www.petmed.com, summarized in the table below.[6] Veterinarians hear these excuses frequently when they approach the touchy topic of ca-nine overweight. Other common excuses include "I don't know what to

TOP 10 OWNER EXCUSES FOR PET OBESITY
1.   But she only eats "this much"!
2.   But he's always hungry.
3.   But food is the only thing that makes him happy.
4.   She'll starve.
5.   He's so old already. I want him to live the rest of his life fat and happy.
6.   I can't bear to know she's suffering from hunger.
7.   He refuses to walk.
8.   It's my family's fault.
9.   Whenever he loses weight, everyone tells me he's too thin.
10. My pets have always been chunky and they have never died early.

do about it," "I tried a special food once and nothing happened after a week," and "he keeps eating the cat's food."

Overweight pets often slow down in their daily activities. They may play less, have trouble going upstairs, or have difficulty jumping into the car or onto their favorite couch. Some may even have difficulty grooming. These signs are often attributed to aging or arthritis. While this may be true, it also can be attributed to weight gain.

Other signs include panting excessively even after mild exercise, slowing down or sitting down during walks, and heat intolerance in the summer. There are several reasons to explain a decrease in activity, such as arthritis, living in a small apartment, or being confined after surgery. In such cases, the amount of food should be decreased to compensate for the lack of exercise.

Your pet's appetite and behavior

A pet who keeps looking for food constantly is rarely a fit one. Begging for food or treats is also a problem. The random eating of treats in pets has the same results as snacking in people: it all adds up. Interestingly, a study entitled "People and Pets Exercising Together" showed that begging behavior did not increase when dogs were fed a weight-loss food. Owners typically commented that their dogs had more pep and were anxious to go out to play or go for a walk.[7]

One sure way to be tempted by begging eyes is to allow your dog to be in the room when you are eating. Veterinary behaviorists actually discourage this. In the wild, the leader of the pack eats first. Others eat next. You should therefore keep your dog away from the table while you eat. Send him outside. Close her up in a different room or in her crate. Once you are done eating, then you can feed your dog. It is not cruel, it's just common sense, and one easy way to resist the temptation to overfeed your pet.

Dogs gain weight when they are allowed to hang around when a baby is fed. Perched in a high chair, babies often throw as much food on the floor as they put in their mouths. If you allow your dog to play vacuum cleaner, it may save you time, but it will slowly create weight gain. This factor is not limited to babies. If your teenager doesn't feel like eating your home-made lasagna, you know where it will end up.

Another precaution is to make sure that your dog doesn't eat the cat's food behind your back.

It is also important to consider the size of treats you give to your pet. Compare these equivalents for a twenty-pound dog and an average-sized woman:[8]

- Giving one small cookie to a dog is similar to you eating a hamburger or a two-ounce chocolate bar.
- Giving one ounce of cheddar cheese to a dog is similar to you eating 2 1/2 hamburgers or two two-ounce chocolate bars.
- Giving one hot dog to a dog is similar to you eating three hamburgers or two two-ounce chocolate bars.

Giving a treat after dogs relieve themselves may be a good way to train puppies, but once training is over, the "potty" treats should be over. If you must give a treat, choose one that is calorie-free (ice cubes) or low in calories (a piece of apple, celery, carrot, broccoli, or green bean). There are also some commercial light treats available.

Your pet's diet

A dog's proper caloric intake depends on its activity level: a couch potato shouldn't eat as many calories as an agility champion. It also depends on breed, reproductive status (spayed, neutered, or intact), metabolism, weight, and many other criteria.

Here are some basic guidelines for a dog's daily intake with an ideal weight:

- 10-pound dog: 300 calories per day.
- 20-pound dog: 500 calories per day.
- 50-pound dog: 1,200 calories per day.

"Free choice" feeding, that is, leaving food accessible at all times, increases the risk of weight gain. Conversely, feeding a measured amount of food in several meals allows controlling the amount of calories. This does not mean that free choice is always a bad idea. If you only feed the amount of food allowed for the day and resist the urge to refill the food bowl that day, you will achieve the same end result. This, however, is difficult to do with dogs who tend to inhale their food all at once.

Your pet's weight

If you have a purebred dog, it is a good idea to know what the average weight is for its breed. There is a breed weight chart listed in the Resources section of this book. Countless web sites dedicated to specific breeds, as well as the American Kennel Club,[9] can also give you this information. Based on the averages, you can figure out where your pet stands. It is important to note that body weight by itself does not indicate

ACTIVE, HAPPY DOGS AND WEIGHT MAINTENANCE

I have found that the only way to keep my three dogs fit is to keep them on weight loss food in strictly measured amounts. In fact, Sampson, my seven-year-old Labrador retriever mix, needs to be maintained on prescription weight loss food to keep his weight under control.

Maggie, a 12-year-old husky mix, was very overweight at 70 pounds when I adopted her four years ago! Thanks to a strict diet food and lots of exercise, she now weighs 43 pounds. She needs to eat prescription weight loss food to maintain her ideal weight.

Jasmine, my most recent adoptee from a shelter (a three-year-old Labrador-sheltie-schnauzer mix) was relinquished because she was "wild and crazy." In fact, she just needed to be able to run, and she turned out to be a great dog. Now, a 15-20 minute leash walk is a mere warm-up for my dogs. During inclement weather, I cut back their food a little to make up for the decreased activity.

It's not just the food that keeps them fit and happy. It's also the exercise they get. My three dogs run freely while I hike over one to two hours, ideally four times a week.

—Denise, a young woman from Pennsylvania

whether your pet is overweight or not. In dogs, weight is relative. This is why veterinarians rely on other more objective criteria than weight alone.

A pet is considered overweight when its weight is 5 to 20% above the ideal weight. A pet is deemed obese when its weight is more than 20% above the ideal.

Another way to figure it out is to look at the dog's "lean" weight at one to two years of age, or once they are fully grown. Unless they already have a weight issue, that can be considered their ideal weight or baseline.

It gets a little trickier with a mixed-breed dog. You can evaluate the ideal weight if you know or can guess the breeds of the parents. Alternatively, you can run a Wisdom Panel, a DNA test, to identify your mixed-breed dog's ancestry with a simple cheek swab.[10]

Physiological factors and your dog's weight

There are a number of physical risk factors that contribute to weight issues in dogs.

Breed

Breeds at risk for weight problems include Labrador retrievers, shelties, cairn terriers, cocker spaniels, Cavalier King Charles spaniels, dachshunds, basset hounds, and beagles.

Some breeds are considered to be less prone to being overweight, including German shepherds, Doberman pinschers, greyhounds, and other sight hounds. However, any of these breeds can become overweight, as vets see in daily practice.

Age

Excess weight is more likely to occur in middle-aged pets because of decreased activity. Young dogs tend to be naturally more inquisitive, energetic, and active, and are assumed to be less likely to be overweight when fed the proper diet. Around 12 years of age, dogs also tend to be less prone to be overweight.

Sex

Females have a higher incidence of overweight and obesity than males.

Reproductive status

Spaying and neutering increases the risk of weight gain by 20 to 25% because it can lead to an increased appetite or a decreased metabolism. This is why many veterinarians recommend switching to a light diet food after sterilization.

According to Dr. Debra Zoran, a board-certified veterinary internist at the Texas A & M veterinary medical school, research has shown that pets need 1/4 to 1/3 fewer calories after being neutered because of hormonal changes. Preventing weight gain should not be a reason to stop neutering pets: the benefits clearly outweigh the risks, in both males and females. However, Dr. Zoran explains, "a light diet food wouldn't be ideal in very young puppies (2-3 months old) as they are still growing and therefore need a growth food. In these pets, I would recommend cutting back on the amount of food, for example, by 25%, and closely monitoring the weight every few months. Once they are fully grown (and that depends a lot on the breed), then I would switch them to a light diet food."

If a dog is neutered at four to six months of age, you could switch to an adult diet food, or go from free-choice feeding to two or three meals daily with a measured amount of food each time.

Obesity is not inevitable, however, even for a female, spayed, middle-aged dog. It is perfectly possible to overcome these risk factors by adjusting the number of calories to your pet's specific needs.

TOP 10 MEDICAL CAUSES OF WEIGHT GAIN IN DOGS

Hypothyroidism (underactive thyroid gland)
Cushing's disease
Diabetes
Cancer (e.g., a mass growing in the belly)
Fluid build-up (ascites)
Pregnancy
Pyometra (infected uterus)
Feeding a regular dog food to a neutered pet
Drugs (cortisone, phenobarbital, potassium bromide)
Breed or genetics

If your pet has gained weight suddenly or recently, your veterinarian is likely to recommend a physical exam, full blood work, and possibly further testing, such as X-rays or an ultrasound. The first step will be to rule out any medical condition or hormonal imbalance. The chart below includes a partial list of medical causes of weight gain. It is critical to detect these conditions or treat them before a weight-loss program is started.

Behavioral factors and your dog's weight

There are also behavioral reasons for weight gain, which can be trickier to diagnose. Some pet owners give a treat after their pet goes outside to eliminate or before they leave the dog to go to work or to the store. Some give breakfast, such as scrambled eggs or bacon. Some give snacks.

"It becomes a habit for the dog and causes the dog to pester the owner for the treats at those times. This makes it hard for the owner to stop giving the treats to help the dog lose weight. This is most harmful to little dogs. Some dogs learn to exhibit the begging behavior to get more treats and it can snowball into a big problem if the owner gives in," explains Susan Bulanda, a Certified Animal Behavior Consultant.

She adds: "Preventing a dog from begging is the best line of defense. But if the dog has learned to beg, curing it can be hard on the dog's owner as well as the dog. One approach is to provide a specific spot for the dog to lie down and wait for a small (one inch square) piece of meat after the dishes are cleared from the table. Initially, the owner may have to re-command the dog to return to this spot until the dog learns to stay there quietly until the end of the meal.

If the owner cannot do this, then removing the dog from the area, either by putting the pet in another room or a crate until the meal is over, and then giving the dog the tiny reward, may work. However, the owner should be prepared to ignore whines, barks, and other noises of complaint until the dog learns that after the table is cleared the reward will appear."[11]

Some feed human food, such as ice cream and potato chips, indiscriminately. Cheap or poor quality food may lead to scavenging because the dog does not get the nutrients it needs. "This can also become a habit since the dog is self-rewarded for doing it," says Bulanda.

STAR, THE CLEVER SAMOYED

Dogs that "counter surf" and open cabinets can get in trouble by eating foods that are toxic. For example, Star, a 100-lb. Samoyed, decided one day to eat an entire box of brownie mix. It wasn't in plain sight. It wasn't left alone on a counter. No, it was in a cabinet. The thing is, Star had learned to open the cabinet and spin the lazy Susan with his paw.

It wasn't the first time, and since chocolate is very toxic in pets, Chrissy, Star's owner, wisely decided to act. She bought a locking device designed to prevent babies from getting into similar trouble, and placed it on her cabinet handles to prevent this from happening again.

—Phil Zeltzman

She says there are other behavioral reasons to explain overweight, including:

- Resource guarding: A dog may eat another pet's food just so the other pet cannot have it.
- Food competitors: Dogs who are raised in some commercial situations have to fight for their food. This happens when several puppies are fed from one bowl. The puppy never fully gets over the feeling that he cannot get enough food. This can cause overeating or resource guarding.
- Food thieves: All dogs are born scavengers, some more than others. If a dog has the opportunity to steal food from a counter top, it does not take long for it to search for food throughout the house. Some dogs even learn to open doors and cabinets.

The Body Condition Score

There is no question that evaluating whether a pet is overweight is somewhat subjective. It depends on the person's own experience and biases. A simple method is routinely used in veterinary clinics to make the evaluation more objective: the Body Condition Score (BCS). The BCS system is a reliable way to estimate a dog's fat content, as it correlates well with more scientific methods. It is dependable whatever the breed and body type are. You can easily use it to assess your own dog.

You might consider reading this chapter with your dog right next to you. It will be a bonding moment (it mostly involves petting!) and might be an enlightening experience.

The most frequently used part of the BCS evaluation is the rib test. If you flatten your hand and rub it along your pet's chest, you should be able to easily feel the ribs. You should even be able to count the ribs. If you cannot, it is because the ribs are covered with fat. If you can see the ribs, however, you are either looking at a greyhound or your pet is too thin.

There are other ways to examine your dog. Viewed from above, your dog should have a waist. There should be a concave indentation behind the rib cage toward the rump area, like in an hourglass. A straight line from the ribs to the pelvis is a sign that your dog is overweight. Viewed from the side, the belly should be tucked up between the chest bone and the front of the thighs. A straight line in the belly area or a sagging belly is a sign of overweight.

The BCS is based on these evaluations. Vets often log that number at every visit as part of the medical record, next to the weight, the temperature, and the heart rate. Two BCS scales are widely used in the U.S.: one with 9 and one with 5 possibilities. In addition, a 7-point BCS scale, known as the S.H.A.P.E. system (see figure 5), is used in the U.K. It is important to specify which scale is used to avoid any confusion. A dog with a BCS of 5 has an ideal weight according to the 9-point scale, but is obese based on the 5-point scale.

The five-point BCS scale

BCS 1. Skinny dog

The ribs are easily felt, with no fat layer. The tail base is bony with no tissue between the skin and bone. The bones are easily felt with no overlying fat. Dogs over six months of age have a severe belly tuck when viewed from the side, and an accentuated hourglass shape when viewed

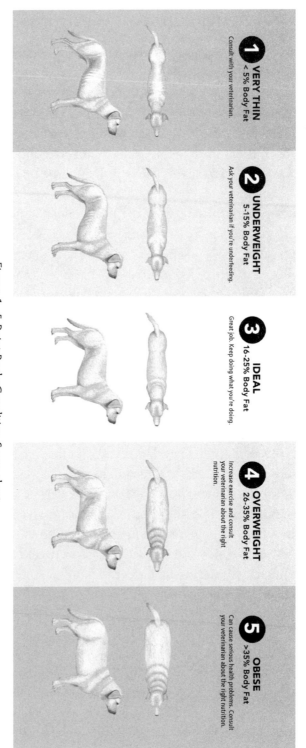

Figure 1. 5-Point Body Condition Score chart.
Reprinted with permission by the copyright owner, Hill's Pet Nutrition, Inc.

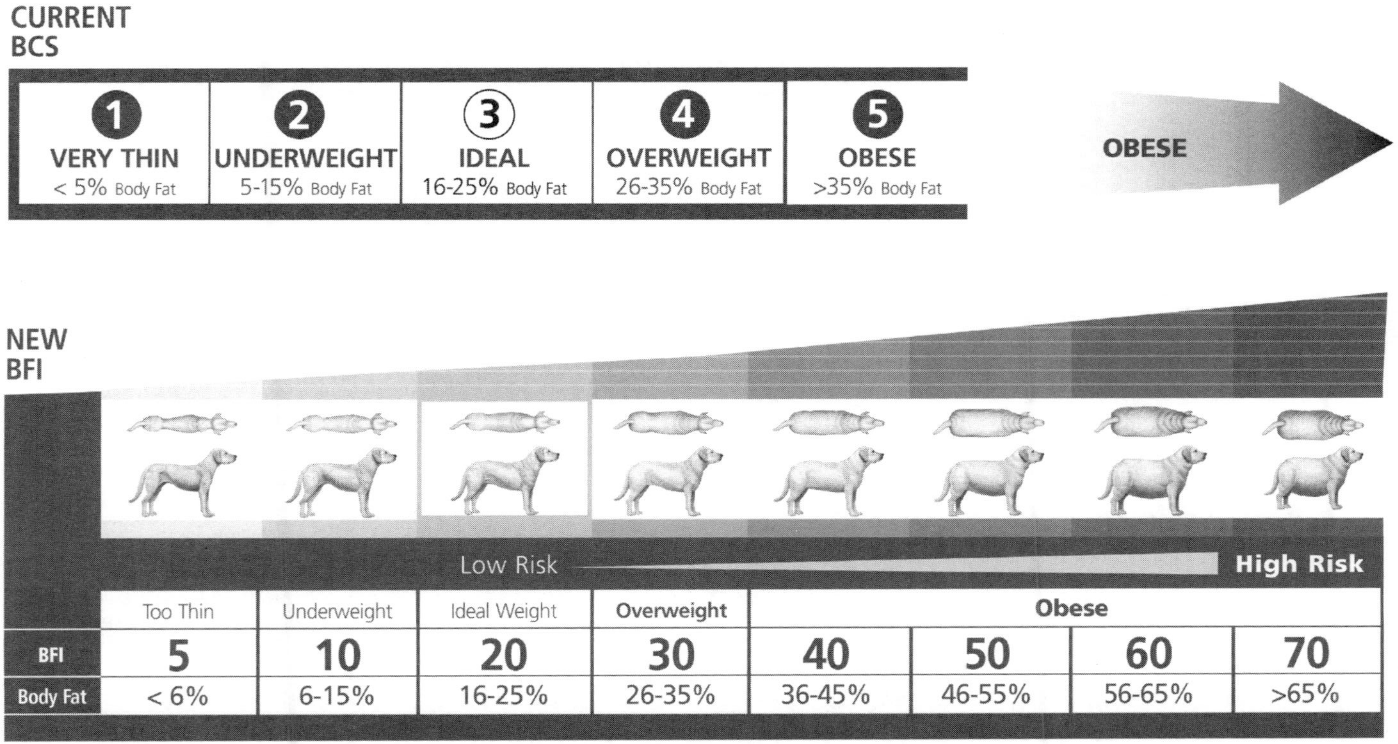

Figure 2. Body Fat Index chart.
Reprinted with permission by the copyright owner, Hill's Pet Nutrition, Inc.

3 Steps To Determine Ideal Weight

Step 1
Weigh the pet.

Step 2
Determine pet's Body Fat Percentage using images & descriptors on the reverse side.

Step 3
Establish ideal weight using this chart.

Ideal Body Weight [lbs]

Current Weight	Body Fat % 20	Body Fat % 30	Body Fat % 40	Body Fat % 50	Body Fat % 60	Body Fat % 70
10	10	8.8	7.5	6.3	5.0	3.8
11	11	9.6	8.3	6.9	5.5	4.1
12	12	10.5	9.0	7.5	6.0	4.5
13	13	11.4	9.8	8.1	6.5	4.9
14	14	12.3	10.5	8.8	7.0	5.3
15	15	13.1	11.3	9.4	7.5	5.6
20	20	17.5	15.0	12.5	10.0	7.5
25	25	21.9	18.8	15.6	12.5	9.4
30	30	26.3	22.5	18.8	15.0	11.3
35	35	30.6	26.3	21.9	17.5	13.1
40	40	35.0	30.0	25.0	20.0	15.0
45	45	39.4	33.8	28.1	22.5	16.9
50	50	43.8	37.5	31.3	25.0	18.8
55	55	48.1	41.3	34.4	27.5	20.6
60	60	52.5	45.0	37.5	30.0	22.5
65	65	56.9	48.8	40.6	32.5	24.4
70	70	61.3	52.5	43.8	35.0	26.3
75	75	65.6	56.3	46.9	37.5	28.1
80	80	70.0	60.0	50.0	40.0	30.0
85	85	74.4	63.8	53.1	42.5	31.9
90	90	78.8	67.5	56.3	45.0	33.8
95	95	83.1	71.3	59.4	47.5	35.6
100	100	87.5	75.0	62.5	50.0	37.5
105	105	91.9	78.8	65.6	52.5	39.4
110	110	96.3	82.5	68.8	55.0	41.3
115	115	100.6	86.3	71.9	57.5	43.1
120	120	105.0	90.0	75.0	60.0	45.0
130	130	113.8	97.5	81.3	65.0	48.8
140	140	122.5	105.0	87.5	70.0	52.5
150	150	131.3	112.5	93.8	75.0	56.3
160	160	140.0	120.0	100.0	80.0	60.0

Ideal body weights are calculated using current weight and body fat index

Figure 3. BFI scoring chart.

Reprinted with permission by the copyright owner, Hill's Pet Nutrition, Inc.

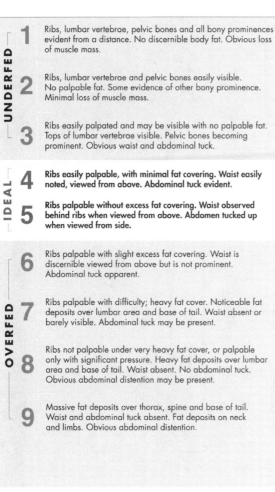

UNDERFED

1 Ribs, lumbar vertebrae, pelvic bones and all bony prominences evident from a distance. No discernible body fat. Obvious loss of muscle mass.

2 Ribs, lumbar vertebrae and pelvic bones easily visible. No palpable fat. Some evidence of other bony prominence. Minimal loss of muscle mass.

3 Ribs easily palpated and may be visible with no palpable fat. Tops of lumbar vertebrae visible. Pelvic bones becoming prominent. Obvious waist and abdominal tuck.

IDEAL

4 Ribs easily palpable, with minimal fat covering. Waist easily noted, viewed from above. Abdominal tuck evident.

5 Ribs palpable without excess fat covering. Waist observed behind ribs when viewed from above. Abdomen tucked up when viewed from side.

OVERFED

6 Ribs palpable with slight excess fat covering. Waist is discernible viewed from above but is not prominent. Abdominal tuck apparent.

7 Ribs palpable with difficulty; heavy fat cover. Noticeable fat deposits over lumbar area and base of tail. Waist absent or barely visible. Abdominal tuck may be present.

8 Ribs not palpable under very heavy fat cover, or palpable only with significant pressure. Heavy fat deposits over lumbar area and base of tail. Waist absent. No abdominal tuck. Obvious abdominal distention may be present.

9 Massive fat deposits over thorax, spine and base of tail. Waist and abdominal tuck absent. Fat deposits on neck and limbs. Obvious abdominal distention.

Figure 4. 9-Point Body Condition Score chart.
Courtesy of Nestlé Purina PetCare Company.

from above. A BCS of 1 indicates that a dog has less than 10% body fat, and is 20% below the ideal body weight. (This score would be equivalent to a BCS of 1 in the 9-point scale.)

BCS 2. Underweight dog

The ribs are easily felt with a minimal layer of fat. The tail base is bony with little tissue between the skin and bone. The bones are easily felt with minimal overlying fat. Dogs over six months of age have a belly tuck when viewed from the side, and a marked hourglass shape when viewed from above. Dogs with a BCS of 2 have less than 15% body fat, and are

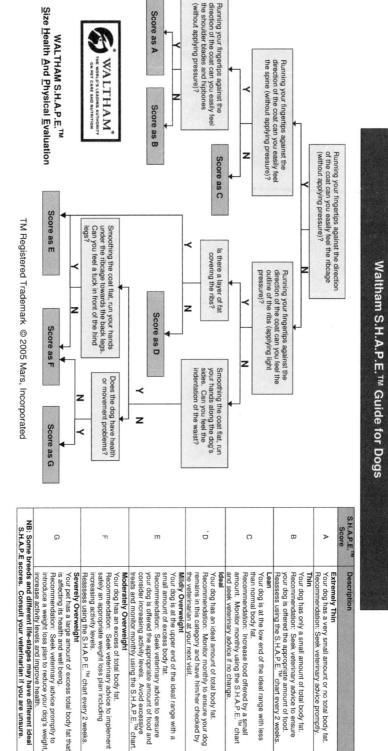

Figure 5. 7-Point BCS / SHAPE guide.
Courtesy of Waltham / Mars Petcare.

10% below the ideal body weight. (This score would be equivalent to a BCS of 3 in the 9-point scale.)

BCS 3. Ideal dog

The ribs are felt with a slight layer of fat. The tail base has a smooth contour or some thickening. The bones are palpable under a thin layer of fat between the skin and bone. The bones are easily felt under minimal amounts of overlying fat. Dogs over six months of age have a slight belly tuck when viewed from the side, and a well-proportioned waist when viewed from above. A BCS of 3 means your dog has 15 to 25% body fat, which is considered ideal. (This score would be equivalent to a BCS of 5 in the 9-point scale.)

BCS 4. Overweight dog

The ribs are difficult to feel with a moderate layer of fat. The tail base has some thickening with a moderate amount of tissue between the skin and bone. The bony structures can still be palpated. The bones are covered by a moderate layer of fat. Dogs over six months of age have little or no belly tuck when viewed from the side. The back is slightly broadened when viewed from above. Dogs with a BCS of 4 have 25 to 35% body fat, and are 10% above the ideal body weight. (This score would be equivalent to a BCS of 7 in the 9-point scale.)

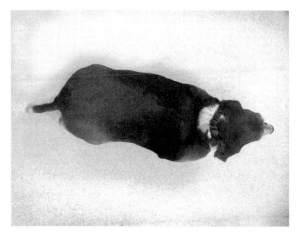

An obese bassett hound.

BCS 5. Obese dog

The ribs are very difficult to feel under a thick layer of fat. The tail base appears thickened and is difficult to feel under a prominent layer of fat. The bones are covered by a thick layer of fat. Dogs over six months of age have a sagging belly, and no waist when viewed from the side due to extensive fat deposits. The back is markedly broadened when viewed from above. Pets with a BCS of 5 have more than 35% body fat, and are 20% above the ideal body weight. (This score would be equivalent to a BCS of 9 in the 9-point scale.)

The 7-point BCS scale uses the following qualifiers to describe dogs: extremely thin, thin, lean, ideal, mildly overweight, moderately overweight, and severely overweight.

The 9-point scale considers dogs with a BCS of 1-3 to be underfed, 4 and 5 to be ideal, and 6-9 to be overfed.[12] The BCS can also be used to follow a trend as a pet is losing weight. It is very encouraging for a pet owner to see their pet going from a BCS of 5/5 to a 4/5 to a 3/5. Then they know the diet food and the extra activity are really working and their efforts were worth it.

A new tool in dogs: The Body Fat Index

It seems that in spite of vets' efforts, dogs' waist lines keep expanding more and more, year after year. Researchers at the University of Tennessee and Hill's Pet Nutrition realized that some overweight dogs had a really hard time losing weight, even when their owners strictly followed feeding instructions.

Expanding on the BCS scale, a new concept has been introduced recently: the Body Fat Index (BFI) scale. This new system describes dogs with a BCS of 4 or 5 in more detail, in order to help identify those dogs that need fewer calories to lose weight effectively.

Let's start with the description of a normal dog, which would have a BFI of 20 (body fat of 16 to 25%). Six criteria are used (see figure 1 for illustrations):

Ribs: slightly prominent, easily felt, thin fat cover.
Shape from above: well-proportioned waist.
Shape from the side: belly tuck present.

Shape from behind: clear muscle definition, smooth contour.
Tail base bones: slightly prominent, easily felt.
Tail base fat: thin fat cover.

An overweight dog might fit in one of five new categories.

BFI of 30 (body fat of 26 to 35%)

Ribs: slightly to not prominent, can be felt, moderate fat cover.
Shape from above: detectable waist.
Shape from the side: slight belly tuck.
Shape from behind: losing muscle definition, rounded appearance.
Tail base bones: slightly to not prominent, can be felt.
Tail base fat: moderate fat cover.

BFI of 40 (body fat of 36 to 45%)

Ribs: not prominent, very difficult to feel, thick fat cover.
Shape from above: loss of waist, broad back.
Shape from the side: flat to bulging belly.
Shape from behind: rounded to square appearance.
Tail base bones: not prominent, very difficult to feel.
Tail base fat: thick fat cover, may have a small "fat dimple."

BFI of 50 (body fat of 46 to 55%)

Ribs: not prominent, extremely difficult to feel, very thick fat cover.
Shape from above: markedly broad back.
Shape from the side: markedly bulging belly.
Shape from behind: square appearance.
Tail base bones: not prominent, extremely difficult to feel.
Tail base fat: very thick fat cover, fat dimple or fold present.

BFI of 60 (body fat of 56 to 65%)

Ribs: not prominent, impossible to feel, extremely thick fat cover.
Shape from above: extremely broad back.
Shape from the side: severely bulging belly.
Shape from behind: square appearance.
Tail base bones: not prominent, impossible to feel.
Tail base fat: extremely thick fat cover, large fat dimple or fold present.

BFI of 70 (body fat of more than 65%)

Ribs: unidentifiable, impossible to feel, extremely thick fat cover.
Shape from above: extremely broad back, bulging midsection.
Shape from the side: very severely bulging belly.
Shape from behind: irregular or upside down pear appearance.
Tail base bones: not prominent, impossible to feel.
Tail base fat: extremely thick fat cover, large fat folds or pads.

Both the BCS and the BFI can help you determine what your dog's ideal weight is. The ideal weight is calculated using the current weight and the body fat index. In turn, knowing the ideal weight helps in feeding what your dog needs to lose weight. Our goal should be to feed what is called the lean body mass (such as the muscles), and not the fat tissue.

Once you and your vet have decided on your dog's BFI, please turn to figure 3, the BFI Scoring Chart, to figure out your dog's ideal weight. Let's take an example. Jake is a plump eight-year-old Labrador with a BFI of 50 and a current weight of 100 pounds. The intersection of these two lines on figure 3 would give Jake an ideal weight of 62.5 pounds, which determines how much he should be fed.

The hope is that by using this new system, we will be able to help more dogs to lose weight and enjoy life more. An added bonus is that we will be able to enjoy our dogs longer, since we know that thin dogs live longer. Below are two testimonials about the potential for weight loss to improve the quality of life for humans and their dogs.

Communicating about overweight and obesity

Once you are aware that your pet is overweight or obese, please talk to your veterinarian about it. To be fair, it is quite possible that vets haven't done the best job of informing their clients that their dog is overweight or obese. There are many reasons for that, starting with lack of time. The list of topics to discuss during the often single, yearly visit to your vet may include the vaccines of the day, external parasite control (fleas and ticks), internal parasite control (intestinal worms and heartworm), results of the physical exam and blood work, tartar on the teeth, maybe a lump noticed in the skin, and so much more. Starting a conversation about excessive body weight and the proper diet food may seem, to

SUSAN AND LINDSAY, A STORY ABOUT LOVE

I have spent the majority of my life at least 100 pounds overweight. Eating was something I did when I felt nervous. Food was a source of comfort from the pain in my life. As a college student, I began a series of attempts to lose the weight and become more physically active. I tried every available diet food program. I never had a problem losing the weight, but could never keep it off because each time I became thinner, I felt the pressure of higher expectations from myself and others.

My life changed when I adopted my first dog, Lindsay, a black Labrador puppy, who was eight weeks old and grew into a gregarious dog with a high energy level. I loved Lindsay as if she were my child, and lavished this love on the dog by giving her many treats each day. I walked Lindsay twice a day and threw tennis balls for her in the back yard for hours each week. But gradually Lindsay became obese like me. She suffered through knee surgery twice, through numerous large fatty tumor removal surgeries, and had problems with her shoulders. My veterinarian tried repeatedly to convince me to stop overindulging Lindsay. But I felt that by depriving Lindsay of treats, I was depriving her of love. Food had been a source of love and comfort for me all of my life.

Gradually, I realized that I was slowly killing both myself and Lindsay. I made the conscious decision to start exercising with Lindsay. Instead of sitting on the porch and throwing the tennis ball, Lindsay and I began to take longer, gradually more vigorous walks. With Lindsay well medicated for her joint problems, she joined me happily and gradually began to lose weight. My commitment to myself and my dog helped me to feel empowered for the first time in my life. Lindsay and I lost our weight together, became more physically fit, and a lot happier. Lindsay saved my life.

—Susan, 52 years old

TULIP'S STORY

Tulip, a very sweet 12-year-old golden retriever, had a cancerous thyroid tumor removed. Three months later, she came back for follow-up chest X-rays, to make sure the tumor hadn't spread to her lungs. The good news: it hadn't spread, and the tumor hadn't come back in the thyroid area. The bad news: Tulip went from 60 pounds at the time of surgery to 76 pounds. In other words, she gained about 25% of her body weight in three months, a huge amount.

Why did this happen? It is very likely that the owners felt bad for Tulip's cancer and overfed her, actually a classic observation. The owners complained that, ever since the surgery, she has more and more difficulty getting up. They thought it was because of the cancer, or the anesthesia, or the surgery, or maybe arthritis.

What these well-meaning owners didn't realize is that they were "killing her with kindness." They had the best intentions in mind. They truly loved their dog and were obviously very dedicated. But they were over-feeding her. A weight-reducing diet food was started. Our cancer-free patient is now losing weight.

—Phil Zeltzman

some vets, like a sure recipe to be late for their next appointment. Vets may also feel reluctant to talk about weight to spare the feelings of the owner, to avoid implying that he or she is a bad caretaker, or to avoid confrontation.

Now that you know where you and your dog are starting off, let's review the consequences of being overweight. In chapter 3, we will examine why it is so important to lose weight.

Notes

1. Finkelstein, E. A., Fiebelkorn, I. C., & Wang, G. (2004). State-level estimates of annual medical expenditures attributable to obesity. *Obesity Research, 12*(1), 18-24.

2. What Your Cholesterol Levels Mean. (2011). American Heart Association. http://www.americanheart.org/presenter.jhtml?identifier=183#HDL

3. What Your Cholesterol Levels Mean. (2011). American Heart Association. http://www.americanheart.org/presenter.jhtml?identifier=183#HDL

4. Understanding Blood Pressure Readings. (2011). American Heart Association. http://www.americanheart.org/presenter.jhtml?identifier=2112

5. German, A. J. (2006). The growing problem of obesity in dogs and cats. *Journal of Nutrition 136*(7), 1940S-1946S.

6. Khuly, P. (2009). Top ten owner excuses for pet obesity. petmd.com blog. http://www.petmd.com/blogs/fullyvetted/2009/february/top-ten-owner-excuses-pet-obesity

7. For a discussion of the PPET study, see Kushner, R. F., Blatner, D. J., & Rudloff, K. (2006). The PPET study: People and Pets Exercising Together. *Obesity 14*(10), 1762-1770; Becker, M. & Kushner, R. F. (2006). *Fitness unleashed! A dog owner's guide to losing weight and gaining health together* (pp. 26-28). New York: Three Rivers Press.

8. Hill's Pet Nutrition, Inc. (2008). Calorie equivalents. Informational brochure.

9. Visit the American Kennel Club's web site at http://www.akc.org.

10. Mars Veterinary. (2011). Wisdom Panel: Discover your mixed-breed dog's ancestry. http://www.wisdompanel.com

11. Email exchange between Phil Zeltzman and Susan Bulanda, Jan. 3, 2010.

12. The Body Condition System was developed at the Nestlé Purina Pet Care Center and has been validated as documented in the following publications: Mawby, D., Bartges, J. W., Moyers, T., et al. (2001). Comparison of body fat estimates by dual-energy X-ray absorptiometry and deuterium oxide dilution in client owned dogs. *Compendium 23* (9A), 70; Laflamme, D. P. (1997). Development and validation of a body condition score system for dogs. *Canine Practice, 22* (July-August), 10-15; Kealy, R. D., Lawler, D. F., Ballam, J. M., et al. (2002). Effects of diet restriction on life span and age-related changes in dogs. *JAVMA, 220*, 1315-1320.

3
Why getting fit is so important
for you and your dog

There are many health issues related to excess weight for both you and your dog, some of which are very serious. This chapter outlines the problems you or your dog may face from excess weight, poor nutrition, or lack of exercise. The good news is that even moderate lifestyle changes can significantly reduce the risk or severity of many diseases. And a gentle, low-impact activity like dog walking is one of the most enjoyable ways to start making these changes.

If you or your dog suffer from joint pain, walking will increase muscle strength around the joints, giving them extra support. Walking brings oxygen to your heart and muscles and increases circulation. Regular exercise can help lower your bad cholesterol and increase your good cholesterol, a one-two punch that lowers the build-up of plaque in your arteries and keeps your blood flowing smoothly. Walking with your dog helps you manage your weight and reduces your risk of type 2 diabetes. Regular physical activity helps you fall asleep faster and deepens your sleep, which in turn reduces stress and boosts your energy levels. Importantly, regular exercise bolsters your immune system, which safeguards against chronic and severe diseases.

Many of these benefits apply to your dog as well. With so much to gain in health and well-being for both you and your pet, it is well worth starting on a dog-walking program. Whatever the condition of you or your dog, walking can ease you both into a higher level of fitness and health.

Weight problems in people

Sixty percent of the U.S. adult population is reported to be overweight, with a BMI over 25, or obese, with a BMI over 30. The lack of physical activity contributing to these problems makes them major health threats. In fact, obesity has been defined as "an excess of body fat sufficient to contribute to disease."[1]

Physical inactivity has been associated with approximately 250,000 deaths annually in the U.S.[2] A recent CDC study showed that only 64% of adults over 18 engage in the recommended level of activity and that 25% actually get no physical activity outside of their work.[3] In another study, rural residents with low incomes were less likely to engage in physical activity than people who live in cities or suburbs.[4] Hours spent watching television among low-income housing residents was associated with fewer steps taken per day.[5] Inactivity is especially common among women, those with low education levels, and the obese.[6]

Stress is a major contributor to the problem of excess weight. Elevated stress hormone (cortisol) levels are one component of a person's allostatic load, which refers to the physiological consequences of chronic exposure to stress.[7] Allostatic load has been associated with overall physical and mental decline as people age. Worse, it accumulates from middle to old age.[8] Long-term stress, which activates the fight or flight response, has been linked to the most common chronic illnesses, including high blood pressure, diabetes, and coronary artery disease. High stress levels have been associated with the life-threatening phenomenon known as metabolic syndrome.[9]

Metabolic syndrome, a collection of risk factors that increase your chances of developing heart disease, stroke, and diabetes, is more common in overweight persons. You are diagnosed with metabolic syndrome if you have three or more of the following:

- A waist measurement of 40 inches or more for men and 35 inches or more for women.
- Triglyceride levels of 150 or higher.
- A high-density lipoprotein level (HDL) under 40 for men or 50 for women.

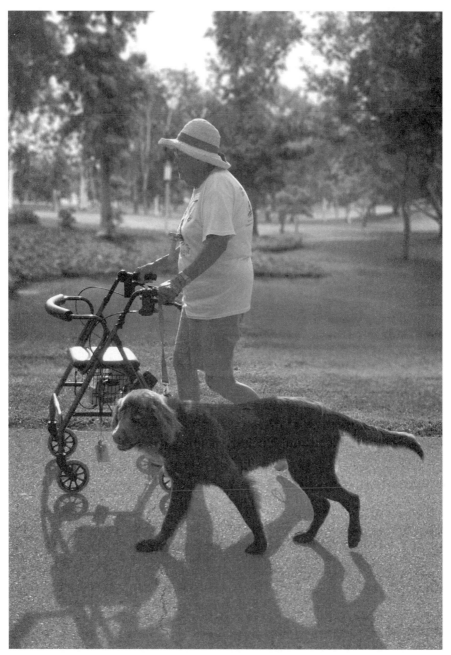

A WAHLAP participant enjoys the evening with her friend.

- Blood pressure over 130/85 or on blood pressure medication
- Fasting blood sugar of 100 or more or on glucose-lowering medication

Weight problems in dogs

It can be more difficult to appreciate the consequences of excess weight in a dog than in a person. For years, veterinarians did not take weight issues as seriously as they should have. We now know better. Overweight in dogs is a major health problem. Not only does it affect their quality of life, but it also affects their longevity. If you love your pet, overfeeding should be the last thing you would ever want to do. In fact, it has been said that overfeeding is just as cruel as starving a dog.

Dr. Debra Zoran, a board-certified veterinary internist at the Texas A & M veterinary medical school, explains, "When a pet eats too many calories, there are only two places these calories can go. Either they are burned through activity, or they are stored as fat. The number of fat cells is typically determined at birth. But beyond a certain size, fat cells can't grow anymore. At that point, new fat cells are created. Fat cells divide into more fat cells.

Once a fat cell is created, it can't be taken away. Fat cells are permanent, although they can shrink in size when calories are burned. So diet and exercise can decrease the size but not the number of fat cells."[10]

All of these extra fat cells translate into extra pounds. Adding seven pounds to a dog who should weigh 35 pounds is the equivalent of an extra 35 pounds on a human who should weigh 175.

The Deadly 13 problems associated with excess weight

The Deadly 13 is our list of the major problems associated with excess weight. Weight loss and physical activity are positive ways to reduce stress and the body's negative responses to it. But what are the costs of remaining overweight? The 13 problems are listed below, and we will examine each in detail.

PET OWNERS' VIEWS ON WEIGHT PROBLEMS

When a pet owner looks at their overweight companion and views it as a normal, healthy weight, I call this the "fat gap." Because of it, our nation's pets will continue to suffer the consequences of obesity. I believe owners have this misperception because they are surrounded by fatter and fatter pets. Twenty years ago, these dogs were viewed as overweight. Today, pet owners view them as normal.

When asked, 33% of dog owners with overweight pets incorrectly identified their pet as a normal weight and 25% of dog owners with obese dogs reported their dog was normal. Interestingly, 33% of small dog owners (less than 23 pounds) thought their overweight dog was a normal weight compared with 41% of large dog owners (over 50 pounds). One notable exception was a study of dachshunds, in which 29% of dachshund owners identified their dog as normal weight when it was actually overweight or obese. In total, 64% of dachshunds in the study were found to be overweight.

Owners of Labrador retrievers and golden retrievers were more likely to claim their dog was a normal weight when it was in reality overweight. And 43% incorrectly identified their overweight retriever as normal while only 33% of small breed dog owners underestimated their dog's weight. In reality, 46% of all Labrador and golden retrievers were determined to be overweight or obese.

The frightening fact is that pet owners are increasingly classifying their overweight pets as "normal," making the problem more difficult to address.

—Dr. Ernie Ward, veterinarian and founder of the Association for Pet Obesity Prevention (www.petobesityprevention.com)

THE DEADLY 13

1. Physical exam issues
2. Degenerative joint disease
3. Surgery risks
4. Anesthesia risks
5. Metabolic diseases
6. Cardiovascular diseases
7. Respiratory diseases
8. Tumors
9. Poor brain function
10. Urinary diseases
11. Skin diseases
12. Pancreatitis
13. Shorter lifespan

1. Physical exam issues

Humans

Overweight and obesity make it more difficult for health care providers to listen to the heart and lungs, make it challenging for them to feel the major internal organs, and make finding a vein difficult to take a blood sample. This means that health problems may be missed until they are very serious.

Dogs

Just as in humans, some of the goals of a physical exam include listening to the heart and lungs and feeling normal and abnormal organs. This is difficult to do in an overweight patient because the veterinarian needs to feel through the fat under the skin and the fat inside the belly. For the same reason, it is more difficult to listen to the heart and lungs.

It is also more challenging to judge dehydration using a skin fold in an overweight dog. Therefore, obesity makes a thorough physical exam difficult at best, and misleading at worst. Diagnostic tests are also more challenging in overweight dogs. Taking a blood sample, performing an ultrasound, obtaining a sample of a lymph node with a needle, or getting a sterile urine sample are all more difficult.

2. Degenerative joint disease

Humans

Joints, particularly the knees, bear the major burden when people carry extra weight. Continual pressure from extra body weight can result in damage to ligaments and tendons as well as breakdown of the cartilage needed to protect joints and make them function without pain. And people with joint pain are less likely to stay physically active. They develop arthritis in these joints, creating more pain, and so the spiral continues. Lack of activity and more immobility leads to loss of muscle mass and muscle strength. The long-term outcome of this spiral is the inability to stay mobile enough to do things that are healthy and enjoyable, so quality of life suffers. There are other health problems that develop from immobility, such as bone breakdown, kidney stones, gout, thickening of the blood, and blood clots in the legs that can lead to strokes or heart attacks. All of these factors combined make overweight and obese people much more likely to be disabled.

Dogs

As in humans, it makes sense that extra weight puts extra pressure on dogs' joints. With this mechanical stress, joint cartilage deteriorates, which leads to arthritis. Moreover, recent evidence in humans and in pets shows that obesity can actually cause arthritis by creating a state of chronic inflammation in the body, which affects joints.[11]

A study followed a group of 48 Labrador siblings for life. Half, the control group, were fed as much food as they wanted. The other half, the food-restricted group, were fed 25% fewer calories. This project led to several published studies over the years, which reached a few key conclusions:[12]

- Thin dogs have less severe hip, shoulder, and elbow arthritis.[13]
- Overweight siblings developed joint problems much earlier, at around six years of age. The thin dogs did not show signs of arthritis on X-rays until they were 12.
- Weight control enabled the thin dogs to live almost two more years.

Besides hip dysplasia (hip arthritis), being overweight can contribute to tears of the anterior cruciate ligament, elbow fractures, and slipped discs. Sadly, there is no cure for arthritis once it is present. Weight loss is a very important step to control this chronic condition. In fact, one study showed that weight loss alone dramatically improved pain from arthritis.[14]

3. Surgery risks

Humans

When an overweight person has an operation, complications are more likely. It is harder for overweight patients to move after surgery, and because of this and other factors, they may be more likely to develop a blood clot in their lower legs. Belly fat may make healing of their operation site more difficult, and make larger people less able to cough and breathe deeply after surgery. This puts them at risk for pneumonia. Day to day strain on their hearts puts overweight and obese people at risk for a heart attack after an operation.[15]

Dogs

It is more difficult to do surgery on an overweight patient. Landmarks are more difficult to feel. Organs and blood vessels are more difficult to see, and therefore complications are more likely. Surgery gloves are constantly greasy and slippery, so using instruments becomes more difficult. Once the surgery is over, it is also more difficult to make a pretty incision on the skin of an overweight patient. Some surgeons actually postpone surgery until the dog has lost weight, in order to improve the outcome. It may be possible in the case of an elective procedure, but it is obviously not an option in an emergency situation. Recovery after surgery is also affected in overweight and obese animals. It is more difficult for them to walk around after orthopedic or neurological surgery.

4. Anesthesia risks

Risks of anesthesia are strikingly similar in humans and dogs.[16] Obese patients face a much more difficult situation from a cardiovascular standpoint than their more slender brethren. The body's cells must be supplied with oxygen and blood to nourish them. Obviously, the greater the total mass of the body, the harder the heart and lungs must work to meet the needs of the cells. Ironically, the very same patients have trouble breathing because they have difficulty expanding their chest. They tend to take quick, shallow breaths. Such patients also tend to have hypercapnia, or too much carbon dioxide in their blood stream, because they can't exhale it properly. This condition actually has a name: the Pickwickian syndrome, or obesity hypoventilation syndrome.

Obesity makes anesthesia more challenging on many levels:

- It is more difficult to place an IV catheter in fatty skin.
- It is more difficult to calculate the dose of anesthesia drugs. In theory, the amount of many drugs should be figured out based on lean weight.
- The longer the surgeon needs to "fight fat," the longer the surgery will be, and therefore the longer the anesthesia will last.

The act of securing the airway for anesthesia is much more complicated in the obese human. The heavier the patient, the smaller the mouth and the shorter the neck, which negatively impacts the anesthesiologist's ability to insert a breathing tube needed to give oxygen and anesthesia gas during the operation.

Overweight patients tend to digest more slowly, that is, the stomach empties more slowly. This can lead to a higher risk of vomiting at the beginning of anesthesia. In turn, vomiting, precisely at the time when the swallowing reflex is decreased, can cause a type of pneumonia called aspiration pneumonia. This means that such patients should fast 12 hours before anesthesia, instead of the standard eight hours.[17]

Simply said, overweight and obese patients don't sleep well under anesthesia. Often, they either sleep too deeply or not deeply enough. Finally, overweight patients may take a long time to wake up after anesthesia. Part of the reason is that they have a hard time "blowing off" anesthesia gases, again because they don't breathe very efficiently.

5. Metabolic diseases

Humans

People who are overweight or obese have a much higher risk of developing non-insulin dependent (type 2) diabetes than those who are not overweight. Insulin is a hormone secreted by the pancreas that is vital to help unlock the body's cells so that they can use glucose (sugar) for energy and growth. In overweight bodies, the cells can become insulin resistant, which means that they do not respond properly to insulin, so they don't get their needed nutrition. Insulin resistance occurs before full-blown diabetes develops. Fat cells are naturally more resistant to insulin than muscle cells, so insulin is not used as effectively as it needs to be.[18]

Gallbladder disease is also more common in people who are overweight. Just as extra weight puts a burden on joints, it also burdens the gall bladder, which releases bile in order to help us digest fats in our diet. Obese people commonly eat more fats than others, so their gallbladder must work harder to keep up with the demand. Obesity also results in a tendency for our cells to become inflamed or irritated, and this can affect the gallbladder as well as other organs.

Dogs

It is often believed that hypothyroidism (underactive thyroid) leads to weight gain in dogs. This may be a myth. Approximately 0.2% of dogs have hypothyroidism, and only half of these dogs are obese. However, about one-third of the canine population is obese. Therefore, some researchers now believe that obesity may actually lead to hypothyroidism.

Whereas fat has long been considered as a storage organ, we now know that just like the thyroid gland, fat produces hormones that communicate with the rest of the body. These hormones can lead to a variety of diseases.

For example, fat produces the hormone adiponectin, which promotes insulin resistance. This in turn can lead to type-2 diabetes in dogs.

Another hormone produced by fat, called leptin, tells the brain when to stop eating. The fatter the animal, the more leptin is produced, until eventually the body becomes resistant to leptin. At this point, the obese pet just doesn't know when to stop eating, and always feels hungry.

Other metabolic consequences of obesity in dogs include increased levels of inflammatory mediators. These substances can cause a number of changes in the body that ultimately lead to reduced quality of life and premature aging.

THE LOVE AND LOYALTY OF LOGAN, THE ENGLISH SETTER

It was easy to convince my sons to hike when they where young, but as they got older they had their own ideas of fun. That is where Logan, an English setter, filled the void. I no longer had to go alone on my adventures.

Eventually, we were going five to seven miles at a time. He loved it! Logan was always ready to go, even in the rain. On hot days, we always walked a trail where there was a stream where he could get a drink. In the winter, we stayed on the south sides of the mountains so it would be warmer.

I know the importance of exercise and have always tried to incorporate it into my life. Sometimes though, I tend to get a bit lax. Having a dog that loves being outdoors and looks forward to his runs makes it hard to get lazy. Logan sits by the door and stares at me. If that doesn't work, he follows me from room to room until I take the hint.

Having Logan's companionship is a blessing. With a crumbling marriage and children away at college, coming home from a tough day at work and being greeted with big wet doggie kisses is heart-warming.

Our walks always make me feel 100% better, no matter what happens throughout the day. Not only is this great exercise for the body, but also for the mind. Keeping up with our routine definitely keeps the pounds off and makes me more content with life. Having a dog is certainly a commitment, but it has so many rewards as well, both physically and emotionally. That is what dogs do to you. They lift your spirits on your worst days. They love you unconditionally, even when you don't like yourself. Their loyalty is immeasurable.

—Christine, a Pennsylvania resident

6. Cardiovascular diseases

Humans

Heart disease commonly occurs in obese people because the heart works harder to pump blood efficiently through the body. Overweight and obese people have higher cholesterol levels. Blood vessels also harden and a build up of plaque forms on their inside walls, so blood clots can form. It is estimated that for every 2.2 pounds of weight gained in adulthood, the risk of heart disease increases by nearly 6% for women and 3% for men.[19] In the U.S., adults often gain ten pounds or more with each decade of life. So they are continually increasing their risk of heart disease. But such weight gain in early and mid-adulthood is often accompanied by high blood pressure and high cholesterol levels.

Dogs

Obesity can affect the function of the heart. There may be changes in heart rhythm and blood volume. It may also cause blood clots and decreased oxygen to the heart. Whether obesity leads to hypertension is controversial in dogs, as scientific studies are conflicting.

7. Respiratory diseases

Humans

Sleep apnea is more common in overweight or obese people because of changes in the throat muscles and the extra work of breathing with added fat across the muscles of the chest and abdomen. Gastric reflux (movement of stomach acid up into the esophagus and throat) is also more common with increased belly fat. This can make it difficult to sleep while lying flat due to heartburn. It can also burn the vocal cords, causing coughing and a hoarse voice.

Getting over a cold or the flu can be more difficult for overweight and obese persons because it is harder for them to cough effectively to clear their breathing passages. Extra weight presses on the chest and abdomen, making it harder to breathe even while healthy. Shortness of breath is common. This, combined with chest and general muscle weakness, makes it difficult to exert for activities such as climbing stairs, moving in a hurry, or walking even short distances.

Dogs

Obesity is a well-known risk factor for the development of tracheal collapse in small-breed dogs. This is a condition where the windpipe (trachea) becomes so flat and narrow that the dog cannot get enough oxygen. Overweight and obese dogs are often out of breath and they tend to huff and puff, even without exercising or when the temperature is comfortable.

8. Tumors

Humans

Breast cancer occurs more often in obese women, and is more likely to come back after treatment in obese women. Obesity affects hormone levels that have been associated with breast cancer. Uterus and colon cancer are also more common among those who are overweight or obese.

Dogs

Obesity may increase the risk of certain benign and malignant tumors such as breast (mammary) and bladder cancer (transitional cell carcinoma). This is true in other species as well. One study concluded that "calorie restriction is the most potent, broadly acting cancer-prevention regimen in experimental (cancer) models in a variety of animal species, including mammals."[20]

Scientists suspect that the same concept applies to humans, that is, that eating less leads to better health and a longer lifespan.

9. Poor brain function

Humans

Obesity occurring in midlife has been strongly associated with dementia in later years. The same has been found for mental functioning. The ability to think clearly and recall information is worse in those who are overweight during midlife or old age. Obese people are less likely to remain actively engaged with life, and may isolate themselves from others because of joint pain, difficulty breathing, and trouble walking. This may lead to depression. Obese people also suffer mistreatment associated with the stigma of being overweight. They receive poorer service in restaurants and retail stores, may be teased, and suffer painful comments made by family, friends, and complete strangers. This makes them more likely to be depressed and to isolate themselves.[21] Often, when obese people are depressed, they console themselves with food. Food may be a lifelong source of comfort for them. This worsens their situation as they eat more and gain more weight.[22]

10. Urinary diseases

Dogs

Obesity can lead to changes in kidney function. Cases of urinary incontinence have been described in obese dogs. Interestingly, the incontinence was resolved when these dogs became thinner. It is also possible that a type of kidney or bladder stone (calcium oxalate) is more common in overweight dogs.

11. Skin diseases

Humans

Overweight and obese people have larger abdomens and breasts because of extra fat stored in those areas. This can cause "fat aprons" which hang down over the rest of the belly. Under these areas, warmth and moisture from sweating can result in yeast infections, which cause extreme itching and burning, and even skin breakdown. Chafing or rubbing of skin areas together (such as on the thighs) can be painful and damage the skin, making other infections possible.

Dogs

Obesity can cause an increase in skin folds, which may predispose to irritation and infection by bacteria. The end result may include scratching, body odor, and skin redness. Some conditions may be due to a decreased ability to groom efficiently, because, simply put, the dog can't turn to reach certain spots. Overweight dogs often have an unkempt hair coat.

12. Pancreatitis

Dogs

Hyperlipidemia is a condition where fat metabolism is abnormal. Some early research indicates that obese dogs have higher levels of cholesterol, triglycerides, phospholipids, and fatty acids. This in turn may lead to pancreatitis, a painful condition of the pancreas which causes vomiting.

13. Shorter lifespan

Humans

Obesity is related to shorter lifespan. In a study of nurses, researchers found that women with a BMI of 22 or less had the lowest risk of death, whereas a high BMI is associated with greater risk of death. Thus, losing weight can not only help our bodies feel better, but also it can also help us to live longer.

Dogs

Recent research shows that being overweight also affects our pets' lifespans.[23] Diseases related to obesity are the fourth most common cause of death in dogs, according to the American Veterinary Medical Association. In the study of Labrador retrievers mentioned above, thin labradors outlived their overweight siblings by an average of almost two years. They died around 13 years of age, versus 11 years for the overweight counterparts. The expression "killing with kindness" is a sad reality.

Another study shows that a high body-fat mass and a declining lean body mass significantly predict death one year prior to dying. On the contrary, having a lean body composition seemed to be very important in health and longevity.[24]

One study concluded that restricting calories is the most effective way to increase lifespan in multiple animal species.[25]

The financial twist: Paying for the suffering of overweight pets

According to a 2007 study by Veterinary Pet Insurance (VPI), "over $14 million was reimbursed to policyholders for conditions associated with obesity." Amazingly, claims related to obesity represented 7% of all medical claims submitted to VPI in 2006.[26]

"Pet owners may think a few extra pounds are acceptable for their pet, but no one finds extra veterinary bills very appealing," explains Dr. Carol McConnell, Vice-President and Chief Veterinary Officer for VPI. "Obesity in pets should be taken seriously by all pet owners. It shortens pets' lives and dramatically increases health risks."

In 2006, the average claimed cost of treatment for obesity-related medical or surgical conditions was $832, up from $713 in 2005 and $702 in 2004. "Pet obesity begins with excessive kindness," says Dr. McConnell. "Food is the primary way some pet owners demonstrate love to their pet. When dog treats and table scraps become signs of affection or behavioral tools, it becomes difficult to effectively regulate a pet's diet."

Jack Stephens, veterinarian as well as founder and president of Pets Best Insurance, agrees. He says, "we know from an insurance perspective that obese pets, like humans, have greater health problems. This is especially true in exacerbating current medical problems, such as arthritis or hip dysplasia. Overweight can also create health problems, such as heart disease, diabetes, and many more. Even with the assistance of pet health insurance paying 80% of veterinary fees, it can still be expensive to treat these. The best thing you can do to manage your pet's health is to control their weight and provide exercise in daily walks or play."

Another veterinary colleague told us that she charges more to perform surgery on an overweight or obese pet than she does to do the same procedure on a lean patient. "It makes sense because surgery will be tougher, it will take longer, and it is riskier," she explains.

Team up with your dog to make changes for the better

Being overweight or obese sadly creates a vicious cycle for people and pets. Joint pain and other illnesses associated with excess weight make it difficult to be active. And a sedentary life can lead to more weight gain, which only makes the problem worse.

It is never too late, however, to make a change for the better for you and your beloved pet. As a team, you can enjoy spending time together as you slowly make your lives more active. You will soon start to feel better and have increased energy for your daily walks.

Together, you can change your lives. Read on to learn how to get started.

Notes

1. Obesity trends among U.S. adults. (2011). Robert Wood Johnson Foundation. http://www.rwjf.org/childhoodobesity/interactive.jsp?id=37. Click Animate to see the yearly progression of obesity in adults. For the definition of obesity, see Finkelstein, E., Fiebelkorn, I., & Wang, G. (2004). State-level estimates of annual medical expenditures attributable to obesity. *Obesity Research, 12*(1), 18-24.

2. Booth, F. W., Gordon, S. E., Carlson, C. J., & Hamilton, M. T. (2000). Waging war on modern chronic diseases: Primary prevention through exercise biology. *Journal of Applied Physiology, 88*(2), 774-787.

3. Physical activity state indicator report. (2010). Centers for Disease Control and Prevention. www.cdc.gov

4. Parks, S. E., Housemann, R. A., & Brownson, R. C. (2003). Differential correlates of PA in urban and rural adults of various socioeconomic backgrounds in the United States. *Journal of Epidemiology & Community Health, 57*(1), 29-35.

5. Bennett, G. G., Wolin, K. Y., Viswanath, K., Askew, S., Puleo, E., & Emmons, K. M. (2006). Television viewing and pedometer-determined PA among multiethnic residents of low-income housing. *American Journal of Public Health, 96*(9), 1681-1685.

6. Physical activity surveillance demographic comparisons. (2007). Centers for Disease Control and Prevention. www.cdc.gov

7. Greendale, G. A., Kritz-Silverstein, D., Seeman T., & Barrett-Connor, E. (2000). Higher basal cortisol predicts verbal memory loss in postmenopausal women: Rancho Bernardo Study. *Journal of the American Geriatrics Society, 48*(12), 1655-1658; Seeman, T., Singer, B., Rowe, J., Horwits, R., & McEwen, B. (1997). Price of adaptation—allostatic load and its health consequences. *Archives of Internal Medicine, 157*, 2259-2268.

8. Seeman, T., & Chen, X. (2002). Risk and protective factors for physical functioning in older adults with and without chronic conditions: MacArthur studies of successful aging. *Journal of Gerontology: Social Sciences, 57B*(3), S135-S144.

9. Sloan, R. P., Huang, M. H., Signey, S., Liu, K., Williams, O. D., & Seeman, T. (2005). Socioeconomic status and health: Is parasympathetic nervous system activity an intervening mechanism? *International Journal of Epidemiology, 34*, 309-315; Kumari, M., Seeman, T., & Marmot, M. (2004). Biological predictors of change in functioning in the Whitehall II study. *Annals of Epidemiology, 14*, 250-257.

10. Email exchanges between Phil Zeltzman and Debra Zoran, July 2007.

11. Kealy, R. D., Lawler, D. F., Ballam, J. M., Lust, G., Biery, D. N., Smith, G. K., & Mantz, S. L. (2000). Evaluation of the effect of limited food consumption on radiographic evidence of osteoarthritis in dogs. *Journal of the American Veterinary Medical Association, 217*(11), 1678-1680.

12. Kealy, R. D., Olsson, S. E., Monti, K. L., Lawler, D. F., Biery, D. N., Helms, R. W., et al. (1992). Effects of limited food consumption on the incidence of hip dysplasia in growing dogs. *Journal of the American Veterinary Medical Association, 201*(6), 857-863.

13. Runge, J. J., Biery, D. N., Lawler, D. F., Gregor, T. P., Evans, R. H., Kealy, R. D., et al (2008). The effects of lifetime food restriction on the development of osteoarthritis in the canine shoulder. *Veterinary Surgery, 37*(1), 102-107.

14. Kealy, R. D., Lawler, D. F., Ballam, J. M., Lust, G., Smith, G. K., Biery, D. N., et al. (1997). Five-year longitudinal study on limited food consumption and development of osteoarthritis in coxofemoral joints of dogs. *Journal of the American Veterinary Medical Association, 210*(2), 222-225.

15. Personal communication to Rebecca Johnson from James Kessel, MD.

16. Personal communication to Rebecca Johnson from James Kessel, MD.

17. Personal communication to Rebecca Johnson from James Kessel, MD.

18. Read more about this in Balentine, J. R. & Mather, R. (2011). Obesity. MedicineNet.com. http://www.medicinenet.com/obesity_weight_loss/article.htm

19. Haffner, S. M. (2006). Relationship of metabolic risk factors and development of cardiovascular disease and diabetes. *Obesity, 14*, Suppl 3:121S-127S.

20. Hursting, S. D., Lavigne, J. A., Berrigan, D., Perkins, S. N., & Barrett, J. C. (2003). Calorie restriction, aging, and cancer prevention: Mechanisms of action and applicability to humans. *Annual Review of Medicine, 54*, 131-152.

21. Konttinen, H., Silventoinen, K., Sarlio-Lahteenkorva, S., Mannisto, S., & Haukkala, A. (2010). Emotional eating and physical activity self-efficacy as path-

ways in the association between depressive symptoms and adiposity indicators. *American Journal of Clinical Nutrition, 92*(5), 1031-1039.

22. Macht, M., Gerer, J., Ellgring, H. (2003). Emotions in overweight and normal-weight women immediately after eating foods differing in energy. *Physiology & Behavior, 80*, 367-374.

23. Kealy, R. D., Lawler, D. F., Ballam, J. M., Mantz, S. L., Biery, D. N., Greeley, E. H., et al. (2002). Effects of diet restriction on life span and age-related changes in dogs. *Journal of the American Veterinary Medical Association, 220*(9), 1315-1320.

24. Lawler, D. F., Evans, R. H., Larson, B. T., Spitznagel, E. L., Ellersieck, M. R., & Kealy, R. D. (2005). Influence of lifetime food restriction on causes, time, and predictors of death in dogs. *Journal of the American Veterinary Medical Association, 226*(2), 225-231.

25. Hursting, S. D., Lavigne, J. A., Berrigan, D., Perkins, S. N., & Barrett, J. C. (2003). Calorie restriction, aging, and cancer prevention: Mechanisms of action and applicability to humans. *Annual Review of Medicine, 54*, 131-152.

26. VPI reimbursed policyholders more than $14 million for conditions associated with obesity. (2007). Veterinary Pet Insurance press release, August 16.

4

Dog walking, step by step

Whether you are a teenager, an adult, or a new or future mom, you will find information tailored to the needs of you and your dog in this chapter. We will also go over some dangers you should know about when walking to protect yourself and your dog as well as some simple precautions to take.

Physical activity and steps per day

The Center for Disease Control recommends that all adults participate in 30 minutes of moderate intensity physical activity (such as brisk walking) each weekday. An easy rule of thumb is that you should be active enough to break a sweat. Your exercise can be done all at once or in 10-minute increments.[1] This is where walking or playing with your dog can help you meet your needed activity in a fun way. Scientists who do physical activity research have determined that 10,000 steps per day is the optimal number to help decrease your risk factors for heart disease and to lose weight. You can keep track of how many steps you walk each day by wearing a pedometer. These simple, digital step counters are inexpensive and can help you to confirm your daily physical activity. Chapter 5 will explain how to choose a pedometer.

Fitness prescription: What people and pets need to stay fit

The nation's experts on health recently developed goals for U.S. citizens of all ages regarding physical activity. Simply stated, they were created to reduce the number of people who do not participate in physical activity and to increase the numbers of adults who participate in "moderate physical activity, preferably daily, for at least 30 minutes per day, and vigorous physical activity 3 or more days per week during 20 minutes each time."[2] Another goal is to increase the number of people who participate in strength, endurance, and flexibility activities. For children and adolescents, the recommendation is "moderate physical activity for at least 60 minutes on 5 or more [out of] 7 days and vigorous physical activity that promotes cardio-respiratory fitness 3 or more days per week for 20 or more minutes per occasion."[3]

Adults' guidelines

The CDC Division of Nutrition, Physical Activity, and Obesity recommends the following:[4]

- 2 hours and 30 minutes (150 minutes) of moderate aerobic activity (e.g., brisk walking) every week and muscle-strengthening activities on two or more days a week that work all major muscle groups (legs, hips, back, abdomen, chest, shoulders, and arms)

or

- 1 hour and 15 minutes (75 minutes) of vigorous aerobic activity (e.g., jogging or running) every week and muscle-strengthening activities on two or more days a week that work all major muscle groups (legs, hips, back, abdomen, chest, shoulders, and arms)

or

- An equivalent mix of moderate and vigorous aerobic activity and muscle-strengthening activities on two or more days a week that work all major muscle groups (legs, hips, back, abdomen, chest, shoulders, and arms).

The charts below outline a program designed by a physical therapist, one for people who are overweight and have not been walking, and one for people who have been walking to some degree. It assumes that you will begin your walking program slowly and progress over a period of time that feels good to you.[5]

WALKING PROGRAM FOR SOMEONE WHO HAS NOT BEEN WALKING	
Weeks 1-3	Walk 10 minutes, 3 days per week
Weeks 4-6	Walk 20 minutes, 3 days per week
Weeks 7-9	Walk for 20 minutes, 5 days per week
Weeks 10-12 and the remainder of the program	Continue to walk for 20 minutes, 5 days per week

WALKING PROGRAM FOR SOMEONE WHO HAS BEEN WALKING	
Weeks 1-3	Walk 20 minutes, 3 days per week
Weeks 4-6	Walk 20 minutes, 5 days per week
Weeks 7-9	Walk for 30 minutes, 5 days per week
Weeks 10-12 and until you are ready to advance to the next level	Continue to walk for 30 minutes, 5 days per week

If you feel that you are unable to start at the lowest level of walking, see how long you feel you can walk and how often, and begin your program at this level. Maintain it for weeks 1-3 and then try to double this time for weeks 4-6. Never force yourself to walk beyond what you feel you can do.

Children's guidelines

The CDC Division of Nutrition, Physical Activity, and Obesity recommends the following:

- One hour of physical activity per day, most of which should be aerobic activity. This can include moderate aerobic activity, such as brisk walking, or vigorous activity, such as running. It should include vigorous aerobic activity on at least 3 days per week. It should also include muscle-strengthening activities, such as gymnastics or push-ups, at least 3 days per week, as part of the 60 minutes. It should include bone-strengthening activities, such as jumping rope or running, at least 3 days per week, as part of the 60 minutes.[6]

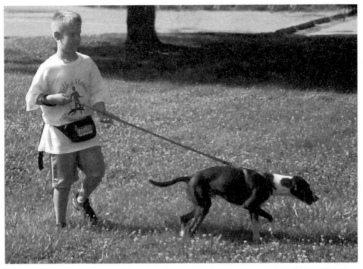

An eager hound leads his young friend through the grass.

Pregnant women and new mothers' guidelines

The CDC Division of Nutrition, Physical Activity, and Obesity recommends the following:

- Healthy women should get at least 150 minutes (2 hours and 30 minutes) per week of moderate aerobic activity, such as brisk walking, during and after their pregnancy. It is best to spread this activity throughout the week.

- Healthy women who already do vigorous aerobic activity, such as running or large amounts of activity, can continue doing so during and after their pregnancy provided they stay healthy and discuss with their health care provider how and when activity should be adjusted over time.

- If physical activity is started during the pregnancy, it should be started slowly and increased gradually over time. During the pregnancy, women should avoid doing any activity that involves lying on their backs or that puts them at risk of falling or abdominal injury, such as horseback riding, playing soccer, or basketball.

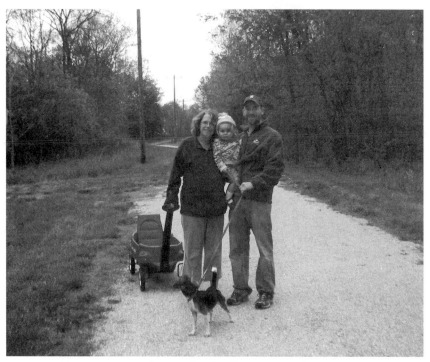

Dog walking makes family time more fun.

- Physical activity does not increase chances of low-birth weight, early delivery, or early pregnancy loss. It's also not likely that the composition or amount of breast milk or the baby's growth will be affected by physical activity.[7]

How much should a dog exercise?

A tired dog is a happy dog, and less likely to look for trouble, such as chewing on your favorite shoes. Yet it is difficult to give general guidelines on how much a dog should exercise. The amount of exercise a dog requires depends on the age, the breed, and even the individual dog's temperament.

As discussed in chapter 1, you shouldn't exercise a young dog too much. Their growth plates, at the ends of their bones, are weaker areas and can lead to deformed bones if they are damaged through too much exercise. Similarly, older dogs shouldn't be exercised as much, but they still should get some activity. It's good for the body and it's good for the mind.

One might think that small dogs need only a little exercise, whereas big dogs need a lot. In fact, small dogs are often bundles of energy that need lots of exercise. Gentle giants such as St. Bernards and mastiffs may, however, be content with shorter walks. Dogs with a flat face may have difficulty breathing, so their comfort level should be closely monitored. Greyhounds and other sight hounds are built for speed, for only short distances. They are sprinters, not marathon runners. And herding dogs typically need more opportunities to walk and run.

A rough rule of thumb is that dogs should exercise at least 15 to 30 minutes each day. This typically means a walk in the morning and a walk at night.

Beyond their breed requirements, each individual will have different needs. For example, one five-year-old Labrador may still behave like a five-month-old, while another Lab of the same age will be rather mellow. Nobody knows your dog as well as you do. With experience, most owners can tell when their dog wants to walk one more mile, and when they're tired and want to go back home.

Walking is an excellent way to get the exercise that we need. Adults are recommended to take 10,000 steps per day. The chart below shows how the number of steps walked per day can give an idea of one's level of activity.[8]

STEPS PER DAY	
Number of steps per day	**Lifestyle**
Less than 5,000	Sedentary
5,000-7,499	Low activity
7,500-10,000	Somewhat active
Over 10,000	Active
Over 12,500	Highly active

Where to walk

The great thing about walking is that it can happen wherever we are—at work, at home, in stores, around neighborhoods, on trails, and in almost any terrain. We can increase our number of steps by choosing to park the car further from our destination, taking the stairs instead of riding elevators, making a long sweep of the hallways at the mall, or investigating what is in the far corner of the library. Trail walking has become very popular in the U.S., as cities and counties recognize the need for people to be more physically active. Such trails usually don't have big hills to climb, so they are a perfect location for people who are just starting out walking or for those with physical challenges. People and dogs of all ages walk on trails. Some trails are paved, while others are surfaced with small gravel. Either are beneficial, but some people prefer not to walk on pavement because it can be hot in summer and offers slightly more resistance on joints—especially the knees and those of the feet.

Issues to consider

Timing of walks

It is best not to walk your dog right after a meal, especially in larger dogs at risk for bloat. Bloat, or gastric dilatation volvulus, is a painful and deadly condition where the stomach becomes full of gas and may twist on itself. Heavy exercise on a full stomach can cause bloating in dogs. Breeds at risk include mostly large dogs such as Great Danes, German shepherds, Weimaraners, setters, retrievers, and standard poodles. You should wait one to two hours before doing heavy exercise after your dog has eaten.

Similarly, walking shortly after eating a meal is not a good idea for people. It may result in side aches or side stitches, which could discourage walking.

Need for water

As we walk, our bodies lose water by sweating (the way our body cools itself) or evaporation. Always carry water and drink before, during, and after walking, and make sure your dog has every opportunity to drink. A dog's cooling ability is actually less efficient than that of a human, so it is important for you to be aware of any signals that your dog is overheated or thirsty. The average person needs an extra 250 ml (about 8.5 ounces) of fluids for every 15-20 minutes of exercise. When temperatures reach 80°F or higher, or in dry climates, significantly more water is needed, such as two to four glasses (16-32 ounces) per hour.[9]

Sunburn

It is important to protect your skin from sunburn while walking. Wearing a sunscreen of SPF 15 or greater is recommended, as is a hat to protect your face and sun glasses to protect your eyes. Some people might benefit from total sunblock lotion. Wearing loose, light colored clothing will help, as will sports clothing especially developed for protecting skin (some fabrics are created for the purpose of blocking the sun's rays).[10]

Dogs can get sunburns as well, and even skin cancer. Especially in dogs with a fair skin and a white hair coat, it is recommended to use doggie sun lotion. Avoid creams with para-aminobenzoic acid (PABA), which can be toxic if licked by a dog.

Risk of heatstroke

Heatstroke is an emergency that happens when our body gets hotter and hotter and is unable to reduce its temperature by sweating. The body temperature can reach 103°F or higher within 10 to 15 minutes. It can happen after over-exercising in a hot or humid environment. In dogs, it can also be due to being locked in a hot car. Either way, this leads to a cascade of very serious conditions which can result in brain damage, organ failure, and death if emergency treatment is not given.

In people, the signs of heatstroke may include red, hot, and dry skin (no sweating), a rapid, strong pulse, a throbbing headache, dizziness, nausea, confusion, and unconsciousness. In dogs, early signs of heatstroke are heavy panting, rapid pulse or heartbeat, dark or bright red gums and tongue, excessive thirst, excessive drooling, followed by lethargy, lack of coordination, seizures, glazed eyes, bloody diarrhea or vomiting, and unconsciousness.[11]

If you suspect symptoms of heatstroke, you should first try to lower the body temperature by moving to a cool area. Cooling procedures should begin before dialing 911 or driving to the hospital.

- You can soak yourself or your pet with cold water, but don't use ice cold water, as it may worsen things. If available, use a fan. It will cool down more efficiently.
- Then dial 911 or drive to the hospital, and get there as quickly and safely as possible.
- If possible, small amounts of water can be offered.

There are some simple, commonsense steps you can take to prevent heatstroke:

- Avoid walking for a long time on hot, humid days.
- Keep your pets indoors except to eliminate.
- Limit outdoor activity to the early morning and late evening, when temperatures are lower.
- Carry plenty of water for you and your dog.

It is important to remember that heat stroke does not only occur in the summer. It's a matter of temperature, not of season.

Hypothermia and frost bite

The opposite of heatstroke is hypothermia. When you are walking in cold weather, you are at risk for developing hypothermia if you are not properly dressed, if your clothing gets wet, or if you stay out too long. This can happen in even cool weather (e.g., 40°F) if you become submerged in cold water or get your clothing wet. When your body temperature drops well below normal, you may shiver, be unable to think clearly, and have difficulty forming words. You may move your hands in a fumbling manner.

Hypothermia is a medical emergency and requires immediate treatment, so activating the emergency response system is necessary. It is important to cover the afflicted person with something warm and get them inside. Never give alcohol to someone in this condition. People often wrongly think that drinking alcohol will keep them warm while they are spending time outside in cold weather. This is absolutely incorrect and puts them at risk for developing hypothermia. If the person is able to swallow, they may be given a warm drink while waiting for the ambulance.

Frostbite occurs when your body tissues actually start to freeze. It happens most often to the toes, fingers, ears, and nose, but can affect the rest of your body as well if you continue to stay out in the cold. Pain in the area is the first sign, but this progresses to numbness, and the area may appear pale, white, or even waxy. Frostbite can make amputation of the affected body part necessary. If no hypothermia is present, the person needs to get into a warm room as soon as possible, preferably without walking on the feet if they are affected.

The same condition can happen in dogs. Hypothermia in dogs is characterized as mild (body temperature of 90-99°F), moderate (82-90°F), or severe (below 82°F). Signs can vary depending on the severity. Mild signs may include lethargy, wobbliness, and shivering. With moderate hypothermia, muscles may be stiff without shivering. With severe hypothermia, many organ systems shut down and the dog may actually appear dead. Emergency treatment should be started by you, and taken over by a veterinarian. It involves warming the patient up, supporting whatever organ is failing, and preventing further heat loss.

Frostbite can also happen to dogs. It most commonly affects extremities such as ears, tail, and toes. The first step is to warm up the dog, but in extreme cases, amputation of the frozen body part may be required.

Drowning

Drowning is a terrible danger you should be aware of if you walk or hike near a body of water. In the winter, frozen ponds and lakes can be misleading. The surface may look safe, but the ice may be thin and may crumble under a person's or a dog's weight.

A LESSON LEARNED

My ten-year-old black Labrador, Mosey and I were at the dog park, where there is a lake. Someone else threw a stick into the lake for their dog to retrieve and Mosey went in after it. Before reaching the stick, she began to go down under water. She could not swim any longer! I ran through the waist-deep water but by the time I reached her, she was under water. I pulled her out and carried her to the shore and she was not breathing. I blew into her nose and after a few tries, she came back to life! Mosey coughed and sputtered but she was alive. I carried her home and took her to see our veterinarian, who prescribed antibiotics to prevent pneumonia. Despite this terrifying experience, she is alive and well today.

—Larry, a Missouri resident

A PREVENTABLE TRAGEDY

Luka, my Husky, and I were walking in early spring around a frozen lake. Luka spotted a duck sitting on the ice and ran after it. To my horror, about 20 yards from shore, she fell through the ice. She began paddling and desperately trying to get up onto the ice, which kept breaking as she tried. After trying in vain to encourage her to keep doing this toward the shore, I crept out onto the ice on my hands and knees but also fell through and could not get to Luka or get out. The rescue team arrived and rescued me, but my dear Luka died. I was hospitalized with hypothermia and survived to grieve the loss of my beloved friend. It was a tragedy that could have been prevented by using one simple device—a leash! Don't take any chances: dogs feel a need to respond to their instincts, and it only takes one time for such a tragedy to occur.

—Danny, an Illinois resident

The damage to the lungs depends on the amount of water that enters the lungs and how quickly medical help is provided. In recent studies, survival in dogs varied between 10 and 60%.[12]

Ideally, CPR should start at the scene for humans and dogs. For dogs this means mouth-to-nose breathing if the animal can't breathe. Wrap the dog in a blanket and take it to the nearest veterinary medical clinic. Call 911 for the human victim and continue CPR until the EMS staff take over. More information about CPR and mouth-to-nose breathing in dogs is available at the Dog First-Aid 101 web site.[13]

Falls

The risk of falling increases as we walk on uneven surfaces and in unfamiliar areas. In 2006, cats and dogs were associated with approximately 1% of the estimated 8 million fall injuries treated in emergency rooms. The falls happened mostly when people were walking or chasing a dog or cat.[14]

One percent is a very small percentage, but we need to be aware that it is very important to do obedience training with our dogs so that they become reliable walking companions. Also, proper shoes (not, e.g., flip-flops) that give good foot support are important to prevent falls.

Safety

Because walking should be enjoyable, it is important to walk in a place where you feel safe. In neighborhoods or parks where safety is an issue, it is always best to walk during daylight hours only and with another person or in a group. Always carry a cell phone in case of emergency.

If a hostile dog comes up to you and your dog while you are walking, walk faster and keep your dog very close to you. Keep your dog from engaging with the hostile dog. Do not scream at or look the hostile dog in the eye. Do not wave your arms or make any movement toward the dog. Ignore the hostile dog and keep walking fast. The hostile dog may keep going if it sees that you are not paying attention to it. If it bites you, try to keep walking toward your destination and call for help. If the hostile dog attacks your dog, do not reach for the hostile dog's head or collar to pull it off of your dog. Instead, get hold of a back leg and pull. This will put the dog off-balance and it should get off of your dog. Quickly let go of the leg and get yourself and your dog away. If the dog knocks you down and is attacking you, "roll into a ball" and "be still like a log." The dog will lose interest in you and leave. Then get medical help immediately and report the stray dog to the local animal control officer.

Snake bites

At best, non-poisonous snake bites can cause a nasty or infected wound. At worst, poisonous snake bites can kill dogs as well as people. If you plan on hiking in an area where snakes are prevalent, you should know how to identify them. Telling the health care team which type of snake bit you is very important. Don't try to kill the snake: it is pointless and you might end up bitten again.

You should be aware that there is a rattlesnake vaccine for dogs. If you are interested, you may want to ask your family veterinarian about it. It is difficult to know how well the vaccine works. There may be some cross-protection with your local rattlesnakes. You also might want to consider enrolling your dog in rattlesnake avoidance training. Dogs end up learning to recognize the smell of the snake and will avoid them if properly trained.

As far as treatment is concerned, a bite is a true emergency. There are various ways to treat a bitten patient, including an antivenin, depending on the severity and location of the bite.

Poison ivy and poison oak

"Leaves of three, let them be" is the old adage that applies to poison ivy and poison oak. Not everyone is allergic to the oils contained in these two "evil" plants. However, to those who are allergic, the raised, red rash, straw-colored liquid weeping from the rash, and extreme itching will be all too familiar. For some, if the oil even comes into minimal contact with skin, a severe reaction occurs within hours. Others can touch the plant with bare hands without being affected. It is important to know what these two plants look like in order to avoid them.

When trail walking, the best protection for people who are allergic to poison ivy is to wear long pants and long sleeves. The clothing must be handled carefully when it is removed so any poison ivy oil on the fabric does not come into contact with skin. Commercially prepared lotions to prevent the oil from entering the skin may be applied before going out for a walk. After contacting poison ivy, it is important to wash the areas thoroughly and quickly after contact. The oil must be removed from the skin or the reaction will occur.

Dogs are believed to be fairly resistant to poison ivy, but they can inadvertently transmit the toxin to a person by contact. If your hands, arms, or legs touch your dog's soiled hair, you may then get poison ivy rash.

Should your dog's skin become irritated, a bath may help. You can protect your own skin by wearing gloves. For trail walking with your dog, if you are allergic to poison ivy, it is important not to handle your dog until its hair coat has been either shampooed or thoroughly wiped down with wet soapy towels.

Ticks

When walking in fields or wooded areas, bringing home ticks is a real possibility. Ticks can transmit a number of diseases, both in dogs and people. The most well-known is Lyme disease, but there is also Rocky Mountain spotted fever, ehrlichiosis, babesiosis, tularemia, and a few others. Ticks can also transmit a toxin during a blood meal that causes tick paralysis in dogs.

If you are in an at-risk area, you should inspect yourself thoroughly, especially your legs and hair. Also inspect your dog carefully after a walk to make sure no ticks are hiding anywhere.

Information is widely available online about the less common tick-borne diseases, so let's talk about the most common one, Lyme disease. Named for the city of Lyme, Connecticut, in which the disease was first recognized, it has been reported in virtually every state in the U.S.[15]

The fear of Lyme disease came to national attention in the late 1970s when the bacterium causing the illness in people was first identified. The bacterium, Borrelia, is found in many species of wildlife (such as deer) but has found humans and pets to be suitable alternative hosts.

In dogs, intermittent lameness is the most common sign. Kidney failure, neurological problems, and even heart disorders can occur as well. It is important to remember that ticks don't cause the disease. They simply transmit the bacteria which are responsible for it. Prevention is therefore geared toward the ticks, not the bacteria.

There are many ways to remove a tick that is embedded into the skin. One is to wipe the area with alcohol over and underneath the tick. Then use tweezers to get a firm grip on the tick and pull it out. Flush the tick down the toilet or drain. Clean your hands and the area where the tick was with warm soapy water.

Antibiotics (such as doxycycline) can help kill the bacteria that cause Lyme disease. Unfortunately, treatment sometimes fails, leading to longer treatments, more health problems, and higher costs. As an added worry, dogs don't develop any long-term immunity after the illness, opening the door to becoming re-infected again and again.

Fortunately, veterinary scientists have found ways to minimize the risks to dogs and help them avoid the nasty effects of this disease. Many of the topical flea products provide protection against ticks as well, so you can discuss the best plan of action with your family veterinarian. Keeping ticks away from your pets literally can be a lifesaver.

Vaccination of dogs against Lyme disease may also be recommended. State-of-the-art vaccines for dogs have been created and can provide an additional level of protection against Lyme disease. Although Lyme-positive dogs have been found in most U.S. states, vets believe that this disease is fairly regional in nature, and owners should have an open discussion with their family vet prior to requesting the Lyme vaccine.

There is no doubt that ticks cause a creepy reaction in most of us. Keeping yourself and your pets tick-free is possible and can prevent serious illnesses.[16]

Leptospirosis

Leptospirosis is a disease caused by bacteria. People come in contact with the bacteria by being exposed to water or food that has animal urine in it. Sometimes, people think that they discovered a beautiful, clear, clean lake and drink the water, wash a piece of fruit in it, or wash their hands in it. In doing this they are at risk for leptospirosis. The bacteria can even enter the skin through a cut. Some people will show no symptoms, but others will develop a high fever, severe headache, chills, muscle aches, and vomiting. They may also have jaundice (yellow skin and eyes), abdominal pain, diarrhea, red eyes, or a rash. This condition requires medical attention. Untreated, leptospirosis can result in kidney damage, meningitis (inflammation of the membrane around the brain and spinal cord), liver failure and respiratory distress. In rare cases, it causes death. The disease is best avoided by not assuming that water is clean.

In dogs, leptospirosis can be a deadly condition. Luckily, it is easily preventable through a simple vaccination. The bacteria Leptospira can cause damage to multiple organs, especially the kidneys and the liver. Dogs can catch the disease in a variety of ways, including near-stagnant water, muddy areas, or areas where contaminated urine from dogs, rodents, or other wildlife might sit. Avoiding these areas is wise but it may be difficult for a hiker. It is therefore critical to discuss this risk with your veterinarian and to be certain that your dog is up to date on vaccination against leptospirosis.

Foxtails

Foxtail is the nickname given to seeds of several grasses which have tiny barbs or spikelets. The most common plant is Hordeum or wild barley. Foxtails break off easily and can attach to pets' hair and people's clothing. The tiny barbs allow foxtails to only move in one direction.

At best, the foxtail becomes so entangled in the hair that some has to be cut off. At worst, foxtails can enter the ear, the throat, or the skin, and migrate inside the body. There have been reports of foxtails going from a dog's nose or throat to the windpipe, though the lungs, though the diaphragm and to the kidney area, where they caused an abscess!

Inhaling foxtails is hard to prevent. At the very least, if you are in an at-risk area, you should inspect your entire dog carefully after a walk to make sure no foxtails are hiding in the fur and the ears. This is true in all dogs, especially if they have long hair.

Nancy Kay, a veterinary internist and author of *Speaking for Spot: Be the Advocate Your Dog Needs to Live a Happy, Healthy, Longer Life*, writes about foxtails:

> These pesky, bristly plant awns grow in abundance throughout California and are reported in most every state west of the Mississippi. A foxtail camouflaged under a layer of hair can readily burrow through the skin (a favorite hiding place is between toes). Not only is the dog's body incapable of degrading foxtails, these plant awns are barbed in such a way that they can only move in a forward direction. Unless caught early, they and the bacteria they carry either become walled off to form an abscess or migrate through the body causing infection and tissue damage. Once foxtails have moved internally, they become the proverbial needle in a haystack—notoriously difficult to find and remove.[17]

Burrs

Similarly, burrs are seeds covered in hooks which easily attach to fur and clothing. Burrs gave George de Mestral, a Swiss engineer, the idea of inventing Velcro. If you are in an at-risk area, you should inspect your entire dog carefully after a walk to make sure no burrs are hiding in the fur.

To remove them, you should wear gloves to protect your own skin from the sharp burrs. You might be able to separate a burr from hair with a steel comb. Tweezers might also come in handy. If it has become impossible to remove burrs, you may need to carefully use scissors to cut the entangled lock of hair. In some cases, you are better off getting help from your vet or a groomer to clip the matted hair.

During the high season for burrs—summer and fall—you may want to consider using doggie boots to protect your dog's feet from the painful burrs. At worst, burrs can cause abscesses, in which case you should take your dog to the vet.

Dog walking shouldn't be feared, it should be enjoyed. However, it is prudent to be aware of these potential dangers so that you know what to look for. Please keep in mind that some dangers are region specific, so it is a good idea to talk to your family veterinarian about what is truly relevant to you and your dog. For example, porcupines, toads, and other wildlife might be an issue in your area.

Conditioning exercises

Warm-up

Before going on a long walk, you should stretch to decrease the risk of muscle, tendon, and ligament problems. And believe it or not, you can do the same to help your dog! It could be as simple as a five-minute warm-up walk before a longer walk. Stretching should include your major muscles: calves, quadriceps (the muscle in the front of your thigh), and hamstrings. In order to stretch properly, your muscle should feel tight, but never painful. Hold the position for 10 to 30 seconds, and do two to three repeats for each exercise. In the Columbia, Missouri Walk a Hound, Lose a Pound community dog walking program, we use the following stretching sequence:

- Roll the shoulders forward and back five times.
- Reach one arm to the opposite side of the body and hold it there with your other hand on the elbow for 10 seconds. Switch arms.
- Reach one arm up alongside of your ear with your hand touching the shoulder on the same side. Hold the elbow up with the opposite hand for 10 seconds. Switch arms.

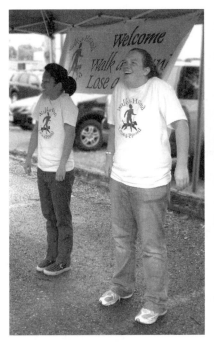

Shoulder roll.

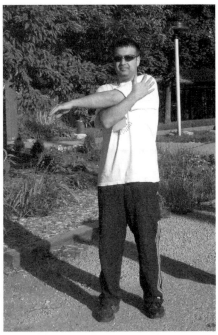

Shoulder stretch.

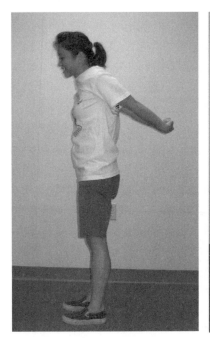

Backward reach.

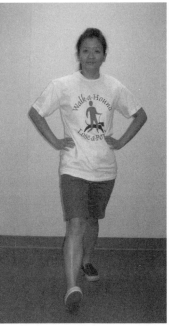

Calf stretch.

- Clasp your hands behind your back and pull your shoulders back for 10 seconds.
- Put one foot out in front of you and lift the toes of that foot, keeping your heel on the ground. Hold for 10 seconds. Switch legs.
- Stand with your feet a little wider than shoulder width, toes facing forward and shift your weight to one foot. Hold for 10 seconds and then shift your weight to the other foot, and hold for 10 seconds.

You can also stretch your dog's joints and muscles. Here are some examples.

- *Back stretch:* While your dog is standing, use a treat to make him or her turn the head toward the tail. Your dog's body will then have the shape of a C. Hold the position, with two to three repeats for each side. A dog reluctant to doing this exercise may have neck or back pain.
- *Shoulder and elbow stretch:* Gently grasp the foot or wrist of your dog and slowly pull the leg forward and upward. Some owners

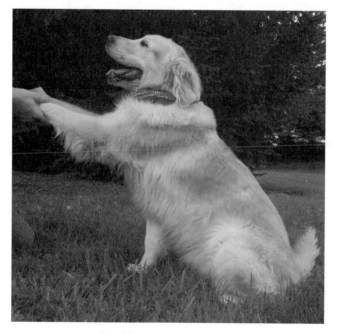

Shoulder and elbow stretch.

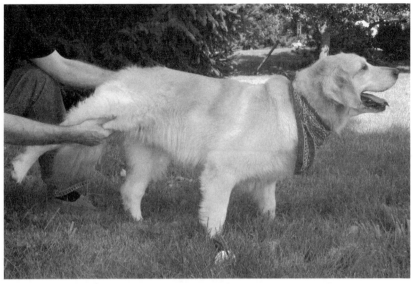

Hip stretch.

may prefer sitting at their dog's side, others prefer to be facing their dog. Hold the position for 10 to 30 seconds, with two to three repeats for each front leg. Resistance to perform this stretch could be a sign of shoulder or elbow pain.

- *Hip stretch:* Gently grasp the knee of your standing dog and slowly pull the leg backward. A normal hip should allow you to extend the leg almost horizontally. Hold the position for 10 to 30 seconds, with two to three repeats for each back leg. This is a common test performed by vets. If the stretched hip causes pain, it can be a sign of hip dysplasia.

If you notice pain during any of these exercises, in yourself or in your dog, do not go on your walk, but check with your primary health care provider or your dog's vet.

Cool down

Similarly, a cool-down period should be allowed before resuming your normal activity. It can be as simple as a five-minute slow, peaceful walk after your walk. After a long hike, the cool-down period could last 10 to 20 minutes.

Successful dog walking

It takes more than avoiding risks to make dog walking fun and beneficial. Humans and canines need to be prepared and be good citizens. This is where leash-walking skills and dog-walking etiquette become important.[18]

Leash-walking skills

Dogs aren't born with leash-walking skills, so you may need to spend some time (re)training your dog to walk on a leash.

For puppies, follow these steps:

- Make your puppy comfortable with a collar. Leave it on in the house, or when he or she is distracted by eating or playing.
- Ignore attempts at getting rid of the collar and reward signs of acceptance.
- Attach the leash to the collar and allow your puppy to drag it around the house, always under supervision.
- Discourage attempts at chewing the leash and reward signs of acceptance.
- After a few days, pick up your end of the leash and start walking around the house.
- If your puppy pulls, fight your instinct. Never pull back. Just stop. Ask him or her to come closer to you and give a reward (a kiss, a hug, or a low calorie treat).
- Resume the walk when your puppy is done pulling.

Your dog also needs to progressively understand that this is a walk, not an opportunity to sniff every smell. So take a short walk first to allow your dog to eliminate. You could use that time to stretch, warm up, and get in the mood. It is also easier to dispose of smelly remains when you are close to home. Afterwards, you should both be in walking mode.

For adult dogs that may have gotten into the bad habit of pulling on the leash, retraining is in order. There are many distractions out there: smells, people, other dogs, squirrels, birds, and butterflies, and dogs think that pulling is the quickest way to get to them.

Here is one possible training plan:

- Go for a walk.
- Every time your dog pulls, stop.
- Encourage your dog to come toward you.
- Reward good behavior with a kiss or a hug.
- Repeat until your dog stops pulling.

Depending on your own preferences, you can add your own commands: "Let's go," "Stop," "Sit," "Heel."

Ultimately, the message you are trying to get across is surprisingly simple:

"Tight leash = we stop."

"Loose leash = we walk."

WALKING RESEARCH PARTICIPANTS COMMENT ON POSITIVE CHANGES

It certainly has made me aware of my weight. My knee doesn't hurt as much because I have been exercising more.

—A 56-year-old married woman who started dog walking

It helped me think about exercise on the weekend.

—A 38-year-old woman troubled with anxiety and depression

Mona was very good on the leash. We talked the whole time we walked. She was very good, a good listener.

—A lady who was happy with her walking companion

It is a wonderful way to show your love of animals.

—A satisfied dog walker

Introducing two dogs on leashes

Introducing two dogs who don't know each other is an art. Susan Bulanda, a Certified Animal Behavior Consultant, says that "the main consideration in allowing two strange dogs to meet while on a leash is to be observant. Be sure to watch both your dog and the approaching dog. Do they look friendly? Does either dog appear to be tense, such as walking stiff legged, tail high and stiff, only waving at the tip? These are signs that a dog may not be friendly. If however, the tail is wind milling, or waving in a complete circle in a relaxed manner, the dog is at ease."[19]

Although it is almost impossible to do, let the dogs approach with a slack leash, but not so slack that you cannot pull the dog away quickly. If the dogs are anxious to meet, let them put the tension on the leash rather than you.

Our behavior consultant continues: "As the dogs sniff each other, watch for mounting behavior, stiffness, direct eye stare, raised hair and freezing behavior. If any of these occurs, gently separate the dogs and let them get used to each other just out of reach.

If they initiate play behavior, such as offering a play bow where the front is low and the rear is raised, then they should be safe together, but until they are fully acquainted, keep a careful eye on them."

More leash tips

It may not be wise to walk a dog and push a stroller at the same time. But if you must do that, at least do not attach the leash to the stroller. If your dog suddenly decides to run after something, it could pull the stroller and flip it upside down, thereby injuring the baby. The same concept applies to bicycling.

Similarly, it is safer to hold the leash in your hand, rather than wrapping it around your wrist or tying it around your waist. Again, if your dog decides to run away, you could lose your balance in the process.

Specialized leashes are available if you want to have your dog's leash attached to your waist. These leashes have safety features including elastic sections to prevent injury should your dog pull.

Dog-walking etiquette

Of course we need to respect others while we walk our dog. This includes respecting people (and dogs) who don't like dogs. Even people who do like dogs don't want a strange dog running up to them (even on

The Ten Commandments of dog walking etiquette

1. Thou shalt keep your dog on a leash.
2. Thou shalt pick up after your dog.
3. Thou shalt avoid dog fights.
4. Thou shalt prevent pulling.
5. Thou shalt allow your dog to drink.
6. Thou shalt check your dog for ticks and burrs.
7. Thou shalt control your dog at all times.
8. Thou shalt be aware of the outside temperature.
9. Thou shalt walk your dog daily.
10. Thou shalt prevent your dog from eating foreign objects (or rolling in them).

a lead), jumping on them, or taking their property. Above are some tips about dog-walking etiquette. If we all adhere to these few suggestions, we can all enjoy our walks even more.

We have explored some of the risks associated with dog walking. In the next chapter, we will present some fun gear for both people and dogs.

Notes

1. Physical activity for everyone. (2010). Centers for Disease Control and Prevention. http://www.cdc.gov/physicalactivity/everyone/guidelines/adults.html

2. Physical activity for everyone. (2010). Centers for Disease Control and Prevention. http://www.cdc.gov/physicalactivity/everyone/guidelines/adults.html

3. How much physical activity do children need? (2010). Centers for Disease Control and Prevention. http://www.cdc.gov/physicalactivity/everyone/guidelines/children.html

4. Physical activity for everyone. (2010). Centers for Disease Control and Prevention. http://www.cdc.gov/physicalactivity/everyone/guidelines/adults.html

5. Personal communication between Rebecca Johnson and Marybeth Brown, 2004.

6. How much physical activity do children need? (2010). Centers for Disease Control and Prevention. http://www.cdc.gov/physicalactivity/everyone/guidelines/children.html

7. Healthy pregnant or postpartum women. (2010). Centers for Disease Control and Prevention. http://www.cdc.gov/physicalactivity/everyone/guidelines/pregnancy.html

8. Tudor-Locke, C. & Bassett, D. R. (2004). How many steps/day are enough? Preliminary pedometer indices for public health. *Sports Medicine, 34*(1), 1-8.

9. Exertional rhabdomyolysis and acute renal impairment—New York City and Massachusetts, 1988: Water requirements during physical activity. (1990). *Morbidity and Mortality Weekly Report (MMWR), 39*, 751-756. http://www.cdc.gov/mmwr/preview/mmwrhtml/00001812.htm

10. Skin Cancer: Prevention. (2010). Centers for Disease Control and Prevention. http://www.cdc.gov/cancer/skin/basic_info/prevention.htm

11. FAQ about extreme heat. (2006). Centers for Disease Control and Prevention. http://www.bt.cdc.gov/disasters/extremeheat/faq.asp.

12. Goldkamp, C. E., & Schaer, M. (2008). Canine drowning. *Compendium, 30*(6), 340-352.

13. Dog CPR may save your dog's life. (2010). Dog First-Aid 101. http://www.dog-first-aid-101.com/dog-cpr.html.

14. Nonfatal Fall-Related Injuries Associated with Dogs and Cats—United States, 2001-2006. (2009). *Morbidity and Mortality Weekly Report (MMWR), 58*, 277-281. http://www.cdc.gov/mmwr/preview/mmwrhtml/mm5811a1.htm

15. The Lyme Disease Foundation. www.lyme.org

16. Visit the Veterinary News Network at www.myvnn.com for short videos on tick-related problems in dogs. Search using the word "tick."

17. Kay, N. (2008). *Speaking for Spot: Be the advocate your dog needs to live a happy, healthy, longer life.* Chicago: Trafalgar Square Books.

18. Westgarth, C., Christley, R. M., Pinchbeck, G. L., Gaskell, R. M., Dawson, S., & Bradshaw, J. W. (2010). Dog behaviour on walks and the effect of use of the leash. *Applied Animal Behavior Science 125*(1), 38-46.

19. Email exchanges between Phil Zeltzman and Susan Bulanda, Feb. 17, 2010.

5

Outfitting for fitness

You can enjoy dog walking in all seasons if you have the proper clothing and equipment to master the elements. This chapter reviews equipment that you may want to consider investing in to optimize your walking. The equipment is for humans and dogs, so you can select which is best for you and your canine walking buddy given the climate that you are walking in. Some gear is essential, so the discussion is categorized according to "must have" or "nice to have."

Before beginning any walking plan, your dog should see a veterinarian and you should see your primary health care provider. People and dogs with health problems or disabilities may have very different requirements.

Must-have clothing for humans

Element-protective clothing

As the Scandinavian saying goes, "There's no such thing as bad weather. There are only improperly dressed people." You need to protect yourself from whatever weather you are going to walk in. This means that in summer, you need light-weight, light-colored, sun-reflective clothing in layers that you can take off as the temperature goes up. Jackets with sleeves and slacks with legs that zip on and off to give you more or less coverage will be versatile in case the weather changes. Long pants will help to prevent you from getting ticks and chiggers if you are walking outside of your neighborhood sidewalks. Shirts that are vented across the back allow for airflow and heat release. A bandana has multiple uses as a perspiration absorber, a coolant when soaked in water, or a bandage if someone is hurt.

A hat to keep sun off of your face and neck is a must to prevent sunburn. Polarized sun glasses will not only protect your eyes, but reduce glare so that you can clearly see obstacles to avoid, or find your dog if he or she is running off lead and gets far afield.

Shoes (including walking sandals) that provide good support and protect your toes from rocks and other obstacles are essential. They come in a multitude of types according to your preference and the terrain that you will be walking in. Ideally, they would be waterproof or at least water resistant.

If you walk at night, you need clothing with reflective strips, or you can wear a reflective vest. You can also buy reflectors that blink. They clip onto your clothing or your dog's collar. Avoid wearing dark clothing at night and never assume that because you can see a car, the driver can see you. Headlights may blind the driver from seeing you and your dog.

In cold weather, it is important to dress in layers so that air is trapped between the layers to keep you warm. Layers can be easily removed when you are too warm. An outer jacket with wind, rain, and snow blocking capacity should help you be prepared for any sudden weather changes. Be aware that in cold climates, low temperatures and low humidity may be exhilarating, but you need to wear warm clothing to prevent frostbite and hypothermia. Long underwear can be purchased that is rated for the temperature range that you expect to be in. It also comes in fabric that wicks moisture away from your skin so that you can stay warm. Outer wear is commonly in dark colors to absorb heat from the sun. Hats and headbands are a must that can be easily removed if you get too warm. Gloves or mittens should be supple enough to allow you to manage the dog's collar, lead, and any other equipment that you carry for the dog.

Waterproof boots will help to ensure that your feet stay warm. Boots or shoes lined with Gore-Tex will allow moisture to escape while preventing water from entering, thus keeping your feet dry. If you walk in icy conditions, it is advisable to put on wiry webs or spikes that fit onto the soles of your boots, or to walk using ski poles. Socks should wick water away from your skin. If you walk in deep snow, gaiters can be purchased that attach to your boots and cover your lower legs with waterproof material.

Must-have equipment

Water containers are a must when you are walking in any weather. If you wait until you are thirsty to drink water, you have waited too long. See our discussion in chapter 4 on the risks of heatstroke and dehydration. There are many different types of water bottles, canteens, and "camels" that enable you to drink even without holding the container in your hands. A camel may be very important if you are hiking in rough terrain. You can carry a pack that will hold your water and other gear, but be aware that it may alter your balance, so practice wearing it fully packed before you go on a lengthy walk. For walking in your neighborhood or on a city trail, even a plastic bottle of water will be fine, as long as you carry enough to last the length of your walk. Dog water bottles come in models that can be used by both you and your dog and easily carried. There are also collapsible cups, inflatable dishes, and many other types of bowls to provide water to a dog. Just make sure you practice using the equipment at home before going on a long hike.

Sunscreen, as mentioned in chapter 4, is a must. Read the label on your sunscreen and don't forget to reapply it if you will be out for longer than its protection length.

Carrying a cellular telephone is a must for walking in any environment. This is especially true if you will be dog walking without any other humans or human-dog pairs. Program speed-dial numbers for emergency help so that you can reach them quickly. Of course, you will need a plan or a phone that allows calls from remote places with limited coverage.

You may also want to carry pepper spray, but be careful of this because if you spray it on a breezy day, it may blow into your face or your dog's instead of where you intend it to go. Also, make sure it is legal in your area.

A first aid kit should at least be kept in your car, even if you choose not to carry it along. You can purchase these at your local drug store. They usually contain bandages for cuts or scrapes, antiseptic cleanser, and other helpful equipment should someone get hurt. They also should be adapted to your particular area: for example, are you more likely to encounter a snake or ticks?

Nice-to-have clothing and equipment for humans

If you are a techy, you may want to invest in a global positioning system (GPS) if one is not already an application on your cell phone. This may be especially important if you are doing wilderness walking, hiking, or trail walking in an unfamiliar area.

A walking stick will be fun to use but also helpful if you are walking on uneven terrain, hill walking, or hiking. It can even be fun to use one when walking on urban trails, and to lean on when you have stopped to talk. It is also helpful in case you encounter an aggressive dog, or if you need to otherwise protect yourself. Walking sticks with seats and water bottle holders are also available.

One useful and motivational tool is a pedometer or step counter, both for you and your dog. The electronic device senses body motion and counts steps over time. Pedometers are not only fun to use, but research shows that they also help to motivate us to walk further and thus get more exercise.[1] Pedometers have been validated by scientific studies, both in people and in dogs. In dogs, they are fairly accurate at a walk, and even more so when the dog trots or runs.[2] They can be found at pet stores and online.

There is a wide range of pedometers available for you and your dog. Some save your steps over a week or a month, others calculate the calories that you have burned, and others just count your steps and need to be cleared each day to start again. Be sure your pedometer has a safety strap that clips onto your clothing or your dog's collar because they are very easy to lose.

In the nice-to-have clothing list, you can purchase clothing that blocks UV rays. This may move into the must-have category if you walk for long periods in climates with a great deal of sun. If you walk regularly or take long walks in challenging terrain such as rocky or hilly areas or on rough trails, you will want to review the wide selection of shoes aimed at each type of terrain and choose some to meet your walking challenge.

The Weather Channel is well known for providing the weather forecast. Their web site also provides tools such as a Walking Calculator, which tells you how many calories you have burned (including by walking your dog) and a Hydration Needs Calculator, which tells you how much you should drink. As of this writing, the way to reach that page from the web site (www.weather.com) is to click on Weather Apps, then Fitness Calculators. You can find a dog walking weather forecast at pet-education.com's Dog Walking Forecast (http://www.peteducation.com/pet-news/). Nuggets of information gathered on the site include:

- A 200-lb. person walking a dog for one hour burns an average of 281 calories.
- Most experts recommend drinking at least a cup of water every 15 minutes of exercise.

In addition to some equipment mentioned above, dogs will benefit from some must-have and nice-to-have gear.

Must-have clothing and equipment for dogs

Leashes, collars, and harnesses

There are countless leashes, collars, and harnesses available for dogs. The simplest combination is a leash and a regular flat leather or nylon collar. Neck collars can cause a number of medical problems to the throat, neck, and spine in small dogs, so it would not be wise to pull firmly on the leash. A collar should be tight enough so that there is no risk of escaping. You should be able to place one finger under the collar to make sure it is tight enough. People with dogs who pull constantly may be tempted to use a chain slip collar, a choke collar, or a pinch collar, but they rarely reach the intended goal and can cause some serious trauma. Most trainers have learned to rely on training more than on these devices.

There are also retractable leashes. Some behaviorists and trainers dislike retractable leashes because it is more difficult to control the dog at the other end. The retractable leash also lets the dog think that pulling is acceptable and gets them where they want to be. There have been a number of incidents, some small, some tragic, which have prompted manufacturers to add disclaimers such as: "To avoid the risk of eye or face injury and cuts, burns, and amputations to your body or the body of another person from the leash cord/belt and hook, read and follow these warnings and directions for use before using your leash." A recent headline from ABC News warns, "Family of Girl, 13, Suing After Snapped Leash Caused Severe Eye Injury."

Similarly, some behaviorists and trainers prefer devices such as the Gentle Leader (www.GentleLeader.com). A regular leash attaches to a head collar. When the leash is pulled, the dog's head turns toward you, which is a gentle way to avoid pulling and choking.

Susan Bulanda, a Certified Animal Behavior Consultant, explains: "The head harness works the same as a halter for horses. The leash attaches to the head harness under the chin. When the dog pulls, the device tightens around the muzzle and lets you turn the head. Where the head goes, the rest of the dog will follow. They are much more humane than neck collars for dogs who are too strong for their owners and who are unruly."[3]

There are several competitors on the market. Body harnesses such as the Halti, the Wonder Walker, and the Easy Walk Harness are also appropriate for strong dogs that pull on the leash. When they pull, they will not choke because the harness pulls on the chest, not on the neck, like a regular collar.

Tags and IDs

There are several ways to provide information about your dog, should it get lost: a permanent tattoo, a microchip under the skin, or simple ID tags. Tags should mention the dog's name, your name, your phone number, and your vet's information. Using at least two ways to identify your dog is certainly not extravagant. Your dog should wear a name tag at the very least, but it can easily get lost. A tattoo or a microchip will be a welcome back up. Tens of thousands of dogs get lost each year, so please don't take any chances.

A critical point to remember is that a microchip is only useful if the information is registered with the proper company from which the chip is obtained. Each microchip contains a unique identification number which is linked to your information (name, address, phone number). Likewise, it is important to change your information if you ever move. Veterinary clinics, shelters, the police, and animal control officers all have microchip readers. Also, be aware that you may need a dog license or a rabies tag in your area.

Nice-to-have clothing and equipment for dogs

Clothing

Clothes are not only meant for dogs owned by movie stars. There are sun-reflecting jackets, raincoats, winter coats, and reflective gear for night use.

Foot pad care

Dogs' foot pads are not as tough as they look. They are quite fragile, and cracks and wounds are often difficult to heal. Pads can be cut by sharp objects and perforated by thorns. In the winter, ice and snow can be tough on foot pads. In addition, road salt and ice melter can cause drying and cracking of the pads.

If you walk in the snow, long hair between food pads should be clipped by a groomer or a technician at your vet's clinic, so that it doesn't cause an accumulation of snow under the feet. Snow, ice, and salt should be rinsed off at home with warm water. Don't forget to gently dry the feet afterward. Carefully inspect foot pads and between the toes to check for sores.

In the summer, hot sand, rocks, or tarmac can cause painful burns on the foot pads. If burns occur, you should wash any open wound with clean, running water. A temporary, loose bandage can be applied until you can take your dog to your veterinarian. Preventing injuries is even better. This typically involves training your dog to wear booties. You also might want to consider trying some products sold with claims to harden foot pads.

Equipment checklist for you

- Clothing appropriate for the season
- Bandana
- Hat
- Sun glasses
- Shoes or boots appropriate for the season
- Appropriate socks
- Reflective gear
- Gloves, mittens
- Ski poles or walking stick
- Spikes for snow boots
- Water supply
- Food
- Sunscreen
- First aid kit
- Pepper spray?
- Cell phone
- GPS
- Pedometer

Equipment checklist for your dog

- Leash
- Collar
- Harness
- Tag, ID
- Clothing appropriate for the season
- Foot pad care
- Booties
- Pedometer
- Water supply and dish
- Toys
- Food
- Treats
- Bandana
- Sunscreen

- Pooper scooper
- Doggie "backpack"

Help on the Internet

There are countless web sites that can help you get ready. A quick search will yield thousands of links. Below is a short selection.

How to choose gear and clothing

About.com: Gear and Clothing for Walkers
   http://walking.about.com/od/gear/Gear_and_Clothing_for_Walk
   ers.htm

How to choose a pedometer

About.com: Before You Choose a Pedometer
   http://walking.about.com/cs/measure/bb/bybpedometer.htm
Pedometer Reviews
   http://www.pedometer-review.com/pedometer-resources/choosing-
   a-pedometer.htm
Walkinginfo.org
   http://www.walkinginfo.org/faqs/answer.cfm?id=1216

Notes

1. Tudor-Locke, C. & Bassett, D. R. (2004). How many steps/day are enough? Preliminary pedometer indices for public health. *Sports Medicine, 34*(1), 1-8.

2. Chan, C. B., Spierenburg, M., Ihle, S. L., & Tudor-Locke, C. (2005). Use of pedometers to measure physical activity in dogs. *Journal of the American Veterinary Medical Association, 226*(12), 2010-2015.

3. Email exchanges between Phil Zeltzman and Susan Bulanda, March 2010.

6

Hate walking?
Here are other great activities with your dog

What can you do if you hate plain walking? There are many other ways to exercise with your dog. Let's discuss a few fun activities that will get you and your dog exercising together. Check out the list below, "Sixteen fun activities to do with a dog," to find one that you and your dog can enjoy. The activities are grouped by intensity, from low impact to more intense. All can be done with your own dog or a loaner dog, such as a friend's or neighbor's dog or one from a local animal shelter.

If your concern is that weight loss is too slow with walking, you have several options: you can increase the distance or the duration, add resistance, or speed up. Increasing distance or speed is easy. To add resistance, you can walk (or run) uphill, swim, or choose from the activities detailed below. But please be patient. Unless you and your dog are already well trained, we suggest that you start with reachable goals, and build up from there. Weight gain didn't happen overnight, so don't expect weight loss to magically occur instantly either. This doesn't happen except in misleading advertising. Other low-intensity activities, such as hide and seek, stair walking, hill walking, hiking, or wading can be altered to increase the intensity by increasing your speed. Be sure to increase speed gradually. It is important to avoid the "weekend warrior" syndrome for you and your dog so that you are not tired and painful the day after doing any of the activities listed.

SIXTEEN FUN ACTIVITIES TO DO WITH A DOG

Activity	Recommendations for Success
Animal-Assisted Activity (visiting people in hospitals, schools, nursing homes)	You and your dog must be registered showing that you are both prepared (check www.deltasociety.org to find out how to become trained and registered)
Taking your dog shopping at the pet store and walking the entire store	Your dog must behave obediently on a nonextendable lead
Hide and seek	Hide a toy and let your dog find it
Stair walking	You can do this inside or outside
Hill walking	
Hiking	
Wading on the beach or in shallow water	
Playing fetch	Be sure not to stand in one place, or only your dog is getting exercise!
Playing tag—chasing your dog and having your dog chase you	Hold your dog's favorite toy to motivate your dog to play
Agility	Take classes with a dog trainer
Jogging	Your dog needs to be reliable at "heel" to prevent falls
In-line skating, rollerblading	Same as for jogging
Bicycling	Same as for jogging
Sledding	Your dog can ride with you and "help" you take the sled back uphill
Cross-country skiing	Same as for jogging.
Surfing—swim alongside the dog	Your dog needs lots of practice to feel secure on a moving surf board

For any activity that you do with a dog—even walking—you and your dog need to prepare for success. Always consult your veterinarian and your primary health care provider before starting to exercise. For walking, preparing for success means that you and the dog need basic leash-walking skills so that you can both have fun while getting exercise. For some of the other activities listed, more specialized training may be needed. The most important thing you can do is to prepare yourself and the dog for whatever activity you will do, so that you can both feel secure enough in the activity to enjoy it. The last thing you need is to push yourself or the dog into something that creates stress. The goal is to have fun exercising together!

Animal-Assisted Activity (AAA)

Some of the activities listed in "Sixteen fun activities to do with a dog" need a little explanation. For example, doing Animal-Assisted Activity (visiting hospitals, schools, or nursing homes with your dog) can be extremely rewarding. Scientists have found that when person-dog teams visit with older adults in nursing homes, the loneliness that the residents feel decreases a great deal.[1] Visiting in facilities even helps the staff who work there to feel less stressed, and to be more likely to talk to one another and to the patients or residents.[2] Children who are hospitalized have been found to have less pain and stress when they receive dog visits.[3] So doing AAA can help many people in different situations. But taking your dog to do these visits can also benefit you and your dog. You will be walking—sometimes a lot—as you go from room to room in a hospital taking your dog to visit. You will also see the joy on the faces of people of all ages who may be comforted, distracted, and just loved by your dog. Many people who start doing AAA continue doing it for the lifespan of several dogs because it is so rewarding.

To do AAA, you and your dog must receive special training. You can't just take your dog to a nursing home and expect good results. The Delta Society is the premier, world-recognized source for this training. Their registered Pet Partners make visits to facilities around the world. You can go to their website, www.deltasociety.org, to register for training, buy training manuals, and do the training at home. Then you and your dog are tested by a Delta examiner before you can become registered. The web site shows you when and where workshops and examining sessions are held.

Your dog needs to have mastered basic obedience skills and be able to ignore rough handling, loud noises, strange places, and awkward situations without a negative response. This includes barking, crying, nipping, biting, jumping up, or fear responses such as avoiding people and places (e.g., fear of getting on an elevator), trembling, drooling, urinating, or vomiting. You need to be able to behave professionally in potentially stressful situations, maintain control of your dog at all times, and to read signs of stress in your dog. While most dogs can be trained to become reliable visitors if their owners are willing to work with them consistently, there are some dogs whose personality will not allow them to be good AAA visitor dogs. Dogs who are fearful, very high-strung or nervous, or who have ever bitten a person are not eligible to become Delta Pet Partners. Similarly, some people's personality will not allow them to be good AAA dog handlers. If either you or your dog become nervous in awkward or unexpected situations, or you cannot handle them, then this is not the activity for you.

Shopping

Going shopping can be fun for both you and your dog. Always check out a store first to be sure dogs are allowed to come in. Pet supply stores commonly allow dogs on leads. Some sporting goods and home improvement warehouse stores also allow dogs. While shopping, you must read your dog's behavior to know if it is becoming stressed by the experience. Behavior such as lip licking, drooling, trembling, whining, urinating, or barking may be signs that your dog is stressed out. Look at your dog's face. If you see its mouth is pulled back on both sides, or if it cannot focus long enough to make eye contact with you, it may be stressed. If your dog's tail stays between its legs, its head stays down, or if it pulls to try to leave the store, then it is time to go. As with any new activity, program it for success by starting out with a very short visit. You can increase the length of shopping time over several visits assuming your dog is not stressed by this activity.

Power dog walks

Some creative and fun "power dog walks" have been created by Gunnar Peterson, the famous Beverly Hills-based personal trainer. This may be just what you are looking for to spice up your dog walking. It combines walking with exercises to help you increase your workout while walking. And it's truly a lot of fun. Spice up your dog walks with intervals, dog tag, fetch abs, dog squat tease, and our personal favorite, the fetch races. This is a great way to bond with your dog. There are nine short videos at www.hillspet.com/weight-management/pet-exercise.html as well as descriptions of a few other fun exercises, such as hide and seek.

Games of fetch

Playing fetch deserves a special mention here because many dog owners sit down or just stand there while throwing a ball, stick, or Frisbee for their dog. This defeats the purpose of exercising together! You can include a game of chase or tag in the fetch game by moving quickly toward or away from your dog between rounds of fetch. There are many variations, such as the Chuckit! Ball Launcher and its many creative variations, or a ball in an old sock.

Agility

Agility training provides not only physical activity but also a mental challenge for you and your dog. In agility, dogs run through an obstacle course of teeter totters, tunnels, bridges, and alternating lines of standing posts. The owner runs along with the dog to encourage and reward the activity and read the behavior of the dog. There are agility trials or contests in which dogs and their handlers compete for prizes based on how fast and accurately they go through the obstacle course. It can be a lot of fun for the dog and the handler-owner, but is not something that most dogs can do automatically. It requires training of both the dog and the handler-owner. Here is a website that introduces agility: www.usdaa.com (United States Dog Agility Association). You should find an agility class that fits you and your dog. Often you can find these by asking your veterinarian or by looking online for a class in your area.

More intense activities

There are many ways to describe exercise. Dr. Christine Zink is both a veterinary pathologist and a consultant on canine sports medicine. She likes to distinguish four types of exercises:

- Stretching, suggested in puppies less than six months of age and for the rest of the dog's life.
- Balancing, for the same groups of dogs.
- Strengthening, for dogs six months and older.
- Endurance, for intact dogs over 14 months of age, and spayed or neutered dogs over 20 months.[4]

The reason for the age limits is that growth plates should be closed before continuous endurance exercise. These weaker areas at the ends of the bones close later in spayed or neutered dogs.

An example of strengthening exercise is retrieving. It requires short bursts of activity with periods of rest in between.

Ideal endurance exercises include swimming for 10 minutes and trotting continuously for 20 minutes. Similarly, running or skating next to your dog is a great way to strengthen your dog and yourself. However, trotting does not mean speeding. You could be walking while your dog is trotting, even slowly. Dr. Zink says that any dog can easily learn to trot, sometimes with the help of a trainer. The trot is a gait where only two feet are on the ground at the same time: left front and right rear, or right front and left rear.

If you are going to do some of the more intense activities with your dog (jogging, rollerblading, or cross-country skiing), keep in mind that your dog needs to be trained, just as you do. You must work gradually into these activities so that no one gets hurt. Always consult your veterinarian and your health care provider before you start these activities. The main issue to consider is safety for you and your dog. You must be able to "read" your dog to know if you are pushing it too hard. You must also listen to your own body rather than exercise "through the pain." Refer to chapters 3 and 4 about the risks to avoid while exercising with your dog. Avoid assuming that your dog can run as long as you can. Just like people, dogs that are not used to running can become short of breath, injure a muscle or joint, or get heat stroke because of over-exercising. Watch your dog's behavior. If your dog lags behind, refuses to move on, favors a leg, or can't seem to catch its breath, there is probably a good reason.

Dr. Zink likes to consider three body shapes in the dog world. This might help you choose the appropriate activity for your dog.

- Light-weight dogs with long legs include greyhounds and sight hounds, border collies, some of the lighter Nordic breeds such as the Siberian husky, Doberman pinscher, and Weimaraner. These dogs are designed for endurance or sprints.
- Heavy-set dogs such as bulldogs and pit bulls are built for strength exercises.
- Moderately structured dogs are breeds such as retrievers, Australian shepherds, beagles, and terriers. They enjoy both endurance and strength exercises.

Now you understand that it is not a complete coincidence if huskies run the Iditarod and Australian shepherds herd sheep. Well-trained, working sled dogs can run for eight or ten hours a day, and they love it. They were bred and built to do that!

Dog walking can be a lot of fun, but you can still hurt yourself if you don't take some basic precautions. Many problems can probably be avoided, both in people and in dogs, by a proper warm up. You should stretch before an exercise program. A slow walk with your dog is an easy way to warm up before picking up the pace. Similarly, a cool down period, which can be as simple as a slower walk, is also a good idea.

Dog parks

Dog parks are worth mentioning here because many people are using them to exercise their dogs. But do the right thing and don't just sit and watch the dogs play!

Dog parks are meant as places for you to play together. Too often, people sit and chat with others, leaving the dogs to play with one another. Dogs are pack animals, no matter how well trained they are. Pack animals, when put into a group, need to see who the boss is. They observe each other and play in ways that show the other dogs where they fit in the order—from top dog to lowest dog. Even dogs that do not seem aggressive at home or with dogs that they know may become hostile in this situation. You can observe aggressive behavior starting if you pay

BRILLO, THE ALL-WEATHER DOG

My running partner, Brillo, a three-year-old German wirehaired pointer, is the greatest exercise companion: she never cancels, complains about the weather, or wants to take a short cut. Together we have logged about 3,500 miles, the equivalent of over 130 marathons!

Running with a dog not on a leash is a very risky thing to do. Even the most obedient dog can get side tracked unpredictably and bolt into traffic or into the path of another person. Not everyone is as big a dog fan as you and I, and some people misinterpret a large brown dog hurtling toward them as a serious threat!

I run with a special belt that holds four water bottles (two for me, two for Brillo) and a little Velcro pocket for a small folding dog bowl. When it's time for a water break Brillo gets to go first.

Any responsible dog owner is all too familiar with the daily poop-and-scoop routine. That doesn't change when we run. Brillo usually manages to find the furthest point from any trash receptacle to maximize the amount of time I have to carry the "package."

Every time I run with Brillo, we share some saga by the end, about the hills we conquered, or about the other runners or dogs we encountered or just the joy of being together doing something we both love. Often, we get so busy with our lives that we forget to stop and feel the joy from the simple things around us, like the smell of damp earth after a spring shower or the sight of the first crocus peeking at us, or the nudge on the elbow from a running buddy congratulating us on a good run.

—Diane, an Ohio resident and marathon runner

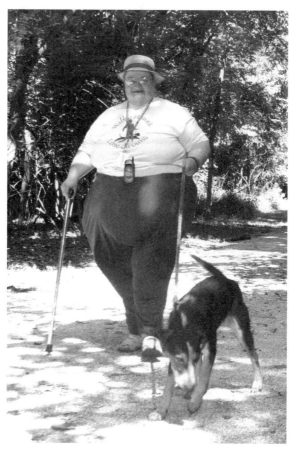

A WAHLAP participant enjoys a summer stroll.

attention. When the hair stands up on a dog's back or when it runs up to another dog, standing face to face with ears up and body tense, then a fight may follow. You should leave the dog park or go to another area, away from the aggressive dog.

You are responsible for your dog's safety. So play with your dog and please pay attention to its behavior. Also be aware of contagious diseases, since your dog will encounter dogs whose vaccination history you don't know. There are many contagious microbes such as parvovirus, Giardia, and the flu virus. Diseases can be caught by getting in contact with feces or urine or simply by being around infected dogs. Your family vet may have some information about which diseases are prevalent in a specific area. Also be courteous and pick up your dog's poop!

Super dog parks

A new generation of dog parks is emerging all around the U.S. Some of these parks are very impressive. They offer play areas, lakes, dock diving boards, wash stations, sand piles, agility courses, fenced areas, and much more. Most are outdoors, but some are now indoors.

The magazine *Dog Fancy* publishes a yearly list of the best dog parks in the nation. We don't want to play favorites, but let's mention a few incredible parks, in Cincinnati, Ohio (www.wagspark.com), Grand Rapids, Michigan (www.shaggypines.com), and Richmond, California (www.ebparks.org/parks/pt_isabel).

Countless other parks throughout the country can be found at the following websites:

- www.dogparkusa.com
- www.usadogparks.com
- www.dogpark.com
- www.hikewithyourdog.com
- www.dogfriendly.com/server/travel/guides/dogpark/dogpark. shtml
- animal.discovery.com/features/dogpark/map/map.html.

Other web sites keep an updated list of local dog parks. For example, Philadelphia dog lovers can visit www.thephillydog.com/?page_id=22.

Camp for people and dogs

People's imagination is without limits. Someone will always come up with a brilliant way to exercise with your dog. For example, Dawn Celapino created Leash Your Fitness (www.leashyourfitness.com), which offers a mixture of boot camp, agility training, and circuit training in San Diego, CA.

Also in several locations in California, there are Thank Dog! Bootcamps (www.thankdogbootcamp.com). Founded by sisters Jamie and Jill Bowers, they are also a great way to exercise and have fun with your dog. Both people and dogs can lose weight there, and you can even borrow a dog if you don't or can't have one (www.thankdogbootcamp.com/ BorrowDog.htm).

Two other camp possibilities are Camp Dogwood, near Chicago (www.campdogwood.com), and Camp Gone to the Dogs in Stowe, Vermont (www.camp-gone-tothe-dogs.com), designed for owners and dogs to exercise, have fun, and relax together. They feature such activities as hiking, agility workshops, dock diving, water play, dancing, and dog massage. You can go for a weekend or longer. You can find other camps throughout the U.S. by searching the internet for "dog camps."

As you can see, there are many opportunities to exercise and have fun with your dog, even if you dislike walking. Pick an activity, try it out, and see if it is a good fit for you and your dog. If not, then simply try another one!

Notes

1. Banks, M., & Banks, W. (2002). The effects of animal-assisted therapy on loneliness in an elderly population in long-term care facilities. *Journal of Gerontology: Biological Sciences, 57A,* M428-M432.

2. Kongable, L., Buckwalter, K., & Stolley, J. (1989). The effects of pet therapy on the social behavior of institutionalized Alzheimer's clients. *Archives of Psychiatric Nursing, 3*(4), 191-198.

3. Sobo, E. J., Eng, B., & Kassity-Krich, N. (2006). Canine visitation (Pet) therapy: Pilot data on decreases in child pain perception. *Journal of Holistic Nursing, 24,* 51-57.

4. Email exchanges between Phil Zeltzman and Christine Zink, June 2010.

7

Get help from the pros

As in many other endeavors, you are much more likely to reach valuable exercise goals if you have a support system. It is helpful to have a friend or a group that can talk over your goals and progress with you. Luckily, there are many ways to find help, live or online.

Help for you

It is important to understand that a lifestyle change, and not a diet or exercise binge, can make the strongest improvement in your health. It is immensely better for you to commit to changing your lifestyle—not to just losing weight for an event, or eating some healthy food for a while. With this in mind, getting expert input will help you develop your plan and take it seriously. So before starting any physical activity or exercise program you need to see your primary health care provider. Describe your existing exercise patterns and any problems that you have had with walking. Also discuss your goals for weight loss or fitness. It is important to be realistic when you set goals. For example, if you have gained a great deal of weight, don't set a goal of returning to the lightest weight of your adult life within six months. Your primary health care provider can help you set a realistic goal by going over your current activity patterns, any physical limitations you may have, and how much weight you need to lose.

Depending on your health and physical activity history, your primary health care provider may want to run some tests, including your cholesterol and triglyceride levels. It is always a good idea to know these numbers. You can request that these blood tests be done if your primary health care provider does not offer them. Remember that you must not eat for at least eight hours before the blood test. If you have a history of any heart trouble, your primary health care provider may want you to have an electrocardiogram (EKG or ECG) to see if your heart is working properly.

It will be important to have your baseline weight taken during this office visit. From there you will be able to track your progress in weight loss and maintenance. During this visit you can also request a consultation with a dietitian or nutritionist to help you analyze your eating patterns and make suggestions for ways to improve your habits.

Speaking of food, you have probably heard of the food pyramid that lists types of foods to eat and in which priority. This pyramid has been recently revised because scientists realized that the previous one-size-fits-all pyramid did not motivate people to eat a healthy diet. The U.S. Department of Agriculture has developed My Pyramid, which provides realistic goals for every person regardless of size, age, or physical health. You can find it at www.mypyramid.gov, with a wealth of information about how to eat healthy foods, where to find affordable, healthy, locally grown food, and how to create healthy meals for you and your family. Important changes in the new food pyramid include:

- A new symbol—a person on the stairs—emphasizing the importance of physical activity.
- Measuring quantities in cups and ounces instead of servings.

The site provides virtually everything you need to help you learn about how to eat a healthy diet. It is an invaluable resource if you're serious about your health. After you click on MyPyramid Tracker, you can enter what you eat and drink for breakfast, lunch, dinner, and snacks. Within minutes, the site tells you:

- How many calories you eat per day.
- How many cups of grains, vegetables, fruit, milk, meat, and beans you consume versus what you should eat.
- How many tablespoons of oil you use per day.

- Your number of calories from extras, which come from solid fats, added sugars, and alcohol. They provide few nutrients but add calories to your total calorie count.

Knowing this information, you can then choose healthier foods and stay on track. And the information is all free of charge.

There are many other ways to keep track, including an iPhone application called LoseIt! (http://www.loseit.com). This free software reportedly enables you to "set goals and establish a daily calorie budget. Stay on track each day by recording your food and exercise and staying within your budget. Enter food and exercise easily using a searchable database. Quickly re-enter foods and meals you've had in the past."

You need a support system

Social support has been found repeatedly in research to be an important factor in maintaining a healthy diet. If you get your whole family involved, you are more likely to have success. Some people find it helpful to join one of the commercial weight-loss programs such as Weight Watchers (www.weightwatchers.com), Jenny Craig (www.jennycraig.

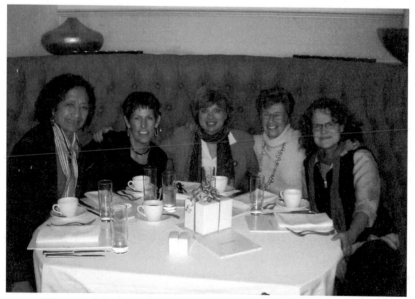

Women of the Woods, five friends who have walked their dogs together for 15 years.

com), or Nutrisystem (www.nutrisystem.com). These programs offer in-person, phone, or online support.

Another option is Take Off Pounds Sensibly (www.TOPS.org), a nonprofit weight-loss support organization based in Milwaukee, WI. Founded in 1948, the group offers chapters located throughout the U.S. and even worldwide. You can join a local group or receive online support.

Another support system is a motivational web site, www.SparkPeople.com. Over 8 million people from over 150 countries have reportedly joined the "SparkPeople movement," so the founders are clearly on to something. You can find a calorie counter, a workout tracker, exercise demonstrations and videos, and even personalized diet and fitness plans.

The message boards allow you to get answers from dietitians and trainers. One of the key features of the site is the support from a team (a "SparkTeam") of online buddies. SparkTeams such as "Walk away the pounds" and "We can do it" allow you to find people with common goals and interests. Being part of a support group can increase your success. And then there's the Success Gallery. The stories are truly inspiring. For example, Aimee, a 21-year-old mom-sales assistant-student, who lost 60 pounds, writes on her own page: "I can participate in all sorts of activities now that I couldn't before, whether it was physical difficulty or just plain shame that held me back."

The most important thing you can do is to select one system that you are comfortable with and stick with it. Your system may be simply to read food labels more carefully and make food choices based on the information found in MyPyramid. That will be much more effective than switching from fad to fad. The critical thing is consistency.

After all, losing weight is pretty simple in theory: you have to eat fewer calories, exercise more, or both. The encouraging thing is that even a slight weight loss of 5-10% of your body weight can be associated with improved blood pressure, blood sugar, cholesterol, and triglyceride levels. But it is important to set realistic goals. They will motivate you if they are short-term and easily accomplished. They are often best if they relate to your eating and exercising behavior, for example, "my goal is to eat a green salad three days this week," "my goal is to walk 15 minutes, four days this week," or "my goal is to stop drinking soft drinks."

There are many tricks that we can use to help us eat less. For instance, when eating out, ask for the "take home" box immediately when your food is served. Then put half of the food into the box and you will eat less during the meal. Put it into the freezer or refrigerator when you get home—no eating a second meal. And you have an extra meal ready to use the next day.

Most restaurants serve helpings that are too large, contributing to our overeating behavior. You can control this by sharing a meal with someone you are dining with. It is fun to decide together what to eat, and even more fun to know you did not overeat. Another tip is to only order an appetizer and a small salad for your meal instead of a whole entrée. But be sure to avoid fried, fat-laden appetizers and choose healthier options such as grilled shrimp, grilled chicken, or a veggie tray with low-fat dip served on the side.

Never supersize a meal from a fast food restaurant. This only adds extra calories that you don't need. Choose from the dollar menu, on which the servings are smaller. Avoid ordering fried foods, and replace French fries or other high-fat side orders with a small salad instead. Read the menu listings of calories for the food you order. Choose the smallest servings of foods with the lowest calorie count. You will be amazed at how quickly you adjust to eating smaller portions of healthier food.

At home, eat meals on a smaller plate. It will look like you have a lot of food but you will be eating less. Remember to keep servings of food smaller than about 2" by 4". Be sure that there is plate showing between servings of food.

Sit down and eat at the table. Slow down your eating by turning off the television and talking with the people at the table with you. Remember what your mom or grandma told you when you were a child, "Take small bites and chew every mouthful of food at least 10 times before you swallow." This gives your brain a chance to catch up with your stomach and tell you that you have had enough food. So don't rush into second helpings.

Try to make mealtime special. Treat yourself by setting the table, turning on some soft music, and lighting a candle. This can prevent you from feeling deprived, as you are eating less food. If the weather is nice, take your meal outside and take time to notice the birds singing, the sounds of the season, and let this atmosphere help your meal be a special time. Never stand at the sink or counter and eat—this may promote eating too fast. Drink a full glass of water before eating and choose water rather than sugary sodas.

Speaking of soft drinks, why not ban them altogether from your life? Do you really need those empty calories or the caffeine in dark sodas? Consuming caffeine may be related to overeating as everything speeds up and your appetite increases. Water is a less expensive and beneficial substitute, which also can enhance weight loss by helping you to feel full.

Unless you have diabetes or low blood sugar, try to eliminate snacks between meals. If you need a snack, eat something healthy like carrot sticks, or some fresh fruit, and drink water between meals. Healthy snacks can help to keep your blood sugar levels even so you don't feel hungry between meals and binge on snacks or overeat during meals.

In making meals at home, avoid prepared meals with high fat and calorie counts. Concentrate on adding whole grains, fresh fruits, and vegetables into every meal. The best part is that healthy food can be as tasty as junk food. There are countless books and web sites that can help you prepare some very easy, very quick, very cheap, and very tasty recipes. One example of an excellent book is *Eat, Drink, and Weigh Less* by Mollie Katzen and Walter Willett, MD, both affiliated with the Harvard School of Public Health. This book will help you learn how to evaluate the benefits of carbohydrates and how to make healthier food. Below is a list of several helpful websites. The first three are very exciting because they are created by the Centers for Disease Control and Prevention (CDC) and contain an incredible array of tips for healthy eating and cooking, with recipes for dishes in virtually every category, from soups to salads to desserts. The fourth web site was created by the famous Mayo Clinic. Some sites include nutrition facts, calorie counts, and the time it takes to make the dishes. This is virtually everything you need to begin healthy cooking and healthy eating—for free.

Websites with healthy recipes and healthy eating tips

- www.cdc.gov/healthyweight/healthy_eating/recipes.html
- www.cdc.gov/healthyweight/healthy_eating/index.html
- www.fruitsandveggiesmatter.gov/
- www.mayoclinic.com/health/weight-loss-recipes/RE00126

Read labels while shopping to make healthier decisions about what you are putting in your body. The USDA estimates that Americans eat over 150 pounds of sugar annually. Most of it comes to us in prepared foods, soft drinks, and sweetened fruit drinks. This is why reading labels is important. When we buy low-fat foods without reading the labels, we may be eating a great deal of sugar that is added to replace the taste of fat. This is why eating "low-fat" food can be very misleading. You may feel good about consciously picking low fat when in fact you are choosing high sugar.

Here is a simple trick to eat less salad dressing while still enjoying its taste. Instead of pouring the dressing on the salad, put a tablespoon of the dressing on your plate. Dip your fork into the dressing as you eat the salad.

Pour out servings of food from bags and boxes and put the bag or box away rather than leaving it on the table, or even worse, eating out of the bag or box. When we eat food out of bags or boxes, we lose track of how much we have eaten and may overeat.

You may want to seek the help of a dietitian as you look for ways to make your eating habits healthier. Your primary health care provider can prescribe a consultation for you, or you can seek out a dietitian yourself. But be careful to seek out a Registered Dietitian (RD). This is a person who has a credential gained by earning a bachelor's degree in dietetics from an accredited college or university. An RD also has to complete at least 900 hours of an internship in a facility supervised by an RD, pass a licensure exam, and complete continuing education in the field every year to maintain the license. An RD knows the science of nutrition and also knows how to counsel people to improve their nutrition. He or she can give you concrete suggestions as to how to improve your eating habits. For more information, you can visit the website of the American Dietetic Association at www.eatright.org. The site includes reviews written by RDs of a long list of popular diets. It also includes valuable nutrition tip sheets on everything from how to read food labels to what constitutes a healthy snack. You can also find an RD in your area with their search system.

You may find "nutritionists" working in health food stores, gyms, or other places who may have a certification as a nutritionist, but no license or formal training in dietetics. This means that they may not be the best source of current and reliable information. Always seek your information from an RD with special training and licensure in dietetics.

Help for your dog

Just as you should see your primary health care provider before starting an exercise program, your dog should see a veterinarian. It can be similar to a yearly checkup, with a complete physical exam and an emphasis on a few key organs such as the heart and the joints.

As discussed in chapter 2, this consultation will allow your vet to check your dog's weight and Body Condition Score (BCS). Remember, there are two main scales for the BCS in the U.S., one where the highest score (obesity) is 5, and one where the highest score is 9. It is important to know which one your vet uses.

It is also a good idea to run some blood work (including a thyroid hormone level) and a urinalysis to make sure all internal organs are working properly. Some undiagnosed diseases can lead to weight gain. Another important part of your discussion with your vet may include something called a diet history: what food you currently feed, how much is fed daily, how many treats, and what types.

Your vet will take this information into consideration when creating a weight-loss plan. The goal often recommended is for your dog to lose 1-2% of its body weight each week.

The exercise program

Have you ever seen an obese wild dog? Probably not. In the wild, wolves, coyotes, and foxes stay in shape by exercising to eat. They have to hunt to survive. Domesticated dogs, however, don't have to work for their food. These days, most grocery and pet supply stores have an entire aisle dedicated to pet food! Some of our dogs' only activity is to walk from the couch to the food bowl, from their dish to the back yard, and from the yard back to the couch. While some of us may envy this stress-free lifestyle, it certainly isn't a healthy or fun way to live.

Dogs are meant to run and play and sniff and explore and play fetch. Many years ago, dogs were actually bred to work, hence their breed names: retriever, terrier, pointer, cattle dog, or sheepdog. When your schedule is so busy that you cannot provide enough exercise, please consider getting outside help. Doggie day camps, dog walkers, and even dog runners may be available in your area. In addition, some vets offer an option which some call "fat camp." Besides leash walks and running, one type of exercise provided is an underwater treadmill. This type of exercise is often provided by a rehabilitation practice at a vet clinic. This is one of the services offered by Dr. Laurie McCauley, a veterinary rehabilitation specialist at TOPS Veterinary Rehab in Grayslake, IL. She states: "By exercising a dog in an underwater treadmill, we are able to stimulate the metabolism without overloading the sore joints of an overweight or obese patient. They typically cannot exercise for very long, so we prefer short, frequent bursts of activity. For example, we might provide three repetitions of five minutes of exercise with two minute long breaks between the repetitions.

Overweight and obese dogs typically do not have strong back legs. A great way for owners to strengthen their dogs' back legs is to make them walk backward and to the side. Of course, we also recommend a strict diet and filling food to complement the weight-loss program."[1]

Dog food changes

It is possible to lose weight by eating a weight-loss diet food but continuing to be a couch potato. Of course, we don't recommend it. A simple and healthier way to look at weight loss is to consider that approximately 50% of results will come from exercise, and 50% from eating fewer calories.

Which dog food to pick is probably one of the most controversial topics in veterinary medicine. There are many options to consider: low fat, low carb, low protein, high protein, raw, the Bones and Raw Food diet (BARF), home-made, store-bought, veterinary clinic-bought, prescription food, dry food, canned food. The diet choices can be quite overwhelming. A recent book, *Chow Hounds*, by Ernie Ward, can help you choose an appropriate food for your dog.[2] We will try to stay away from the controversy and focus on some facts.

Always do a slow transition when you switch dog foods. This will make acceptance of the food easier, and it will lower the risk of diarrhea.

Ten-Day Schedule for Switching to a New Dog Food		
Day	**Amount of current dog food**	**Amount of new weight-loss dog food**
0	100% of current amount	0% of suggested amount
1	90%	10%
2	80%	20%
3	70%	30%
4	60%	40%
5	50%	50%
6	40%	60%
7	30%	70%
8	20%	80%
9	10%	90%
10	0%	100%

Veterinarians typically recommend switching over seven to ten days. Ten days is probably an easier way to do it, as shown above.

A crash diet will provide poor results in dogs just as in people. This concept involves severe restrictions in calories each day, that is, starving the poor dog, in order to achieve rapid weight loss. Unfortunately, the weight lost is often gained back quickly, a phenomenon called the rebound effect. In dogs, a loss of 1-2% of their body weight each week is typically recommended. In people, a steady weight loss of two pounds per week is often recommended.

Most vets agree that cutting the amount of food in half (or by one-third) is not ideal to lose weight. Why? Because while you will obviously lower the amount of calories, you will also decrease the amount of nutrients, including protein, fatty acids, vitamins, and minerals. That is not ideal for weight loss. For example, protein is important to maintain muscle mass. In fact, weight-loss foods are typically richer in protein to promote a lean body condition. So cutting the amount of a maintenance or regular food will starve the dog, which is not considered ideal or humane. Starving your dog will lead to distress, begging, and possibly stealing of food. This is why veterinarians often recommend switching to a weight-loss dog food, which will help your dog lose weight without starving.

A higher-fiber content will make the stomach feel full, a phenomenon called satiety. Because of the higher fiber content of some weight-loss foods, some dog owners notice larger stools. One way to look at it is as an indication that the special food is working. The reason is that fiber is not digested by dogs, and is therefore eliminated.

Fat is an important source of calories, so most weight-loss foods are lower in fat. It makes sense, since fat contains approximately twice as many calories as protein or carbohydrates. A decrease of 25-40% in calories is typical in weight-loss foods.

In fact, there are many ways to design a weight-loss food. It can be high protein, high fiber, low carb or low fat, or any combination thereof. Each pet food company has its own formula that is deemed ideal. Ultimately, what matters (and what works) is to feed weight-loss food that is high quality and balanced yet low in calories and to feed food that your dog actually likes.

Another decision is whether dry food or canned food is better. This depends in part on the dog's preference and the owner's choice. But from a scientific standpoint, canned food is often not as rich as dry food, because calories are diluted by the water content. In fact, canned food contains about 70-80% water.

Choosing a "light" food from your favorite pet store may often lead to disappointing results. It may help maintain a pet's weight, but it rarely seems to help a pet lose weight. They are usually not light enough. Once your dog has an ideal weight, then it may be possible to feed a light food from the pet store or your vet to maintain the weight.

Studies show that dog owners are often overwhelmed by the choices available. Visit any large pet store, and you will see dozens of light dog foods. Even more confusing are the food labels. Some dry foods range from about 200 to over 400 calories per cup. So how are you supposed to choose objectively? In addition, the foods vary widely in price. Dr. Lisa Freeman, a board-certified veterinary nutritionist, comments in an interview: "There is so much information and misinformation about pet foods, it's understandable that people are confused about what to feed their dogs."[3]

The best thing to do is to talk to your family vet or to consider a consultation with a nutritionist. In fact, over 90% of pet owners say they would like to receive pet food recommendations from their vets.

As we have discussed in chapter 2, the cause of pet obesity is occasionally related to genetics, medications, or disease. But ultimately, we need to accept the fact that we are the ones filling our pet's food bowl. So until our pets feed themselves, as they used to in the wild, we are in total control, and we are responsible. It may be tough to accept, but it is the sad truth: when we give our pets too many calories and too many treats, they ultimately pay the price.

Frequency of meals

With an overweight dog on a weight-loss program, it is best to avoid free feeding and instead feed multiple small meals throughout the day. Try to come up with a schedule that fits your lifestyle. For example, you might want to give a small meal in the morning, another one when you come back from work and a third feeding well before going to bed. Avoid feeding just before or right after heavy exercise, as this can cause bloat, a potentially life-threatening condition affecting mostly large breed dogs.

If you are able to go home at lunchtime, you can split the daily amount into four meals. What is the benefit? Digesting and absorbing food requires energy, so it is believed that eating multiple small meals will burn more calories than eating only once or twice.

Treats

Treats are often given to dogs throughout the day, for a number of reasons, and they contribute to the total number of daily calories. What's the big deal with giving a treat to your pet? A treat is proportional to the pet's size and weight. For example, giving a treat to a 20-pound dog (depending on the contents) may be equivalent to a human eating a hamburger.

Treats are often an integral part of the human-animal bond, so banning their use is probably not realistic. They are often allowed, as long as they are part of the daily intake and not given in addition to the allotted food. They typically shouldn't represent more than 10% of the daily food intake. Be especially careful if you use treats to reward a dog in training.

If treats are a must, then at least choose healthy, low calorie treats, either sold in stores or at your veterinary clinic. What is a healthy treat? It could be a piece of carrot, broccoli, green bean (frozen or not), apple or plain rice cake. Alternatively, give a smaller treat: half or a quarter of one. Your dog never took math, and most likely won't even notice the difference! Be sure not to give any treats that are toxic to dogs, such as raisins, grapes, Macadamia nuts, chocolate, or onions.

The best way to provide treats is to take them out of the measured amount of food planned for the day. Again, it is doubtful that your dog will know the difference between an actual treat and a piece of the regular food. It's your love and attention they're after, not a specific type of food.

Table scraps

Table scraps are another controversial topic. They may be acceptable for some dogs. However, there are four main issues with table scraps:

- They can encourage begging, which can become annoying with time.
- They add on to the daily intake of calories, and therefore can lead to weight gain.
- They may change the balance of some nutrients, for example, for a dog on a bladder stone prevention food.
- Fatty foods can cause a painful disease called pancreatitis. This condition of the pancreas causes belly pain and vomiting.

Feeding tricks

To slow down dogs who tend to "inhale" their food, you can spread the food on a cookie sheet or in a muffin pan. Some dogs can be trained to work for their food by using a food ball or a treat ball. These toys are filled with food, and as the dog plays with them, a small piece of food falls out. Again, the food used should be part of the daily calories.

Here is one idea to make sure you are not feeding more than you should. We use this trick every day with our own pets. Place the measured amount of food for the entire day into a special container. The food you use, for actual meals or as treats, is taken from the container as needed. When the container is empty, no more food or treats are allowed for the day. This is helpful when several people, with different work shifts and hectic lives, are involved in feeding your dog. This way, there can be no confusion as to whether someone else fed the dog.

As with any special food, a weight-loss diet food should only be fed to the dog that needs to lose weight. If you have several dogs, make sure that you separate them to feed them individually. Crate feeding or feeding in different rooms are easy ways to do this. They also ensure that there will be no fights during feeding time.

Dog food should be measured, not eye-balled. It is always surprising that some pet owners claim to feed "only two cups a day." When quizzed, it turns out that the "cup" can represent just about anything: a mug, a recycled plastic container, who knows? Dog food is usually estimated in measuring cups, with the understanding that a measuring cup contains 8 ounces.

Weigh-ins and rechecks

Especially at the beginning of a weight-loss program, your vet may recommend recheck examinations every two to four weeks. It is a good time to review the program, make sure that everybody at home is on board and answer any questions you may have. In addition, vets typically recommend weighing your dog monthly to assess the effectiveness of the weight-loss program. This enables you to keep a record of the weight. It will also help determine if you are on track. If your dog is not losing weight as anticipated (1-2% of body weight each week), then it is generally safe to decrease the volume of weight-loss food by 10%. But if you are on track, then it is time to celebrate.

Many vets will provide access to their scale at no charge. Just make sure that someone writes the weight in your dog's medical record.

With a small or medium dog you can easily carry, you can use a regular scale at home. One way to do it is to weigh yourself, holding your dog in your arms. Then put your dog on the floor, without coming off the scale, and weigh yourself. The difference between those two numbers is obviously your dog's weight. And in the process, you just weighed yourself. So you can keep track of your weight and your dog's in the privacy of your own bathroom.

Toward the end of the weight-loss program, rechecks might become more frequent. For example, you may have gone back to the clinic monthly, and now you may need to do it every other week. The reason is that your vet now needs to determine when to stop the weight-loss program and when to start a whole new process: keeping your dog's weight stable and avoiding rebound weight gain. This will typically require a light food as opposed to a weight-loss food. So your vet will generally share some new advice and some new feeding tips once your dog's target weight has been reached.

A weight-loss medication

Slentrol (dirlotapide) is a prescription medication for dogs that works as an appetite suppressant and prevents some of the fat from being absorbed by the body. In fact, 90% of its efficacy is due to appetite reduction and 10% is related to the decreased fat absorption. The end result is weight-loss, at a rate of about 3% per month. Studies conducted with Slentrol showed that almost 98% of the dogs enrolled lost weight, with an average loss close to 12% over four months. However, if habits are not changed, then Slentrol will be a failure. The real secret is to switch to a light diet so that the dog doesn't regain the weight once off the drug. With a true understanding of what went wrong previously (too much food, too many treats, too much people food), success can definitely be reached.

The concept is the same as some medications for people, with a big difference: dogs on Slentrol don't have gas or oily poop. Talk to your family veterinarian to see if your dog is a good candidate. There are a few situations in which it should not be used in dogs, such as liver disease.

Don't forget your dog's joints

An important point to keep in mind when you start a walking program with overweight dogs is that they may have arthritis, whether it is related to obesity or not. To help them walk more willingly and more comfortably, you may want to give some glucosamine and chondroitin sulfate in the form of a joint supplement. Some dog foods provide some glucosamine, but veterinarians often recommend giving some supplements by mouth in addition to what may be in the food. Supplements are not regulated by the Food and Drug Administration, and therefore their quality can vary greatly. Studies show that the amount of glucosamine can be far different from what the label claims. Ask your family vet which brand you can trust.

Nutrition consultation

For multiple reasons, we can only suggest general guidelines for weight-loss food. It is simply impossible to make appropriate blanket recommendations for an overweight three-year-old otherwise healthy Labrador, a plump eight-year-old terrier with diabetes, and a pot-bellied 12-year-old poodle with Cushing's disease.

If you use a commercial dog food and need advice, the pet food company may provide a consultation line. Look for a toll-free phone number on the bag. Be aware that official guidelines by the Association of American Feed Control Officials (www.aafco.org) only allow three descriptors to indicate that a diet dog food might help a dog keep the weight off: "light," "lite," and "low calorie." This means that these foods must meet specific calorie levels set by AAFCO. For example, a "light" or "lite" food should contain 3,100 kilo-calories (kcal) per kilogram of dry food or 900 kcal per kg of wet food.

However, "less calorie" or "reduced calories" only means it that the food has fewer calories than the equivalent product in the same moisture-content category (dry, semi-moist, canned). The label must include the percentage of calorie reduction.

In some situations, for example, if you prefer a home-made meal instead of a commercial food, you may want to consult with a board-certified veterinary nutritionist. "While all veterinarians play an important role in providing nutritional information to pet owners, a board-certified veterinary nutritionist has undergone additional extensive training in veterinary nutrition during their residency. A board certified veterinary nutritionist is a veterinarian who has fulfilled the many requirements to become a member of the American College of Veterinary Nutrition (ACVN), established in 1988."[4]

A list of board-certified veterinary nutritionists can be found at www.acvn.org, the web site of the ACVN. Most nutritionists work at vet schools and in the pet food industry, and a few work in vet hospitals. You can find a list of vet schools which offer nutrition consultations at www.acvn.org by clicking on "Nutrition Resources" at the bottom left. Consultations can be in person or over the phone.

A few board-certified veterinary nutritionists offer online help for a variety of conditions, including overweight and obesity, in exchange for a consultation fee. Such sites include:

- www.petdiets.com, created by Dr. Rebecca Remillard, a nutritionist in Massachusetts. The site can be used by pet owners as well as veterinarians to create individualized homemade diets.
- www.californiapetchef.com, designed by Dr. Meri Stratton-Phelps, a nutritionist in California. Pet owners can get help by phone or email.

Don't go it alone

There is no question that is takes commitment and dedication to help your dog lose weight. But you also need to make sure that everybody in your family has the same goal as you do. Organize a family meeting, and make sure that everybody understands the consequences of obesity for your dog and that you are all committed to helping. The same goes for friends and neighbors, the pet sitter, and anybody who may feed your dog or give it treats.

One study by Pfizer Animal Health showed that one of the top challenges 36% of dog owners face is that there are other people feeding the dog. Once you understand how bad overweight or obesity is for your dog, your next task is to relay the information to your family, friends, and neighbors. If they are not on board, then it is pretty likely that they will undermine your hard work. And ultimately, the big loser will be your dog.

Obviously, readers of this book are true pet lovers, who want to do what is best for their pet. For example, for years, you may have showed your love by giving treats. Honestly, what is greater in life than coming back from a hard day's work, giving a treat to your dog, and seeing this wonderful wagging tail going crazy—surely a sincere expression of happiness?

Yes, what is better in life? Well, a walk to the park may be even better for both of you. In doing this you will be stepping away from a food-centered relationship toward a companionship- and an exercise-centered relationship. But some people need help with this change, as in the story of Mae and Minnow.

Clearly, by walking your dog, you will nurture the unique bond you share. Your dog will benefit from the exercise, and you will too!

Minnow the dog's new zest for life

Mae, the 84-year-old owner of Minnow, a 10-year-old dachshund, was unable to walk Minnow enough because of knee pain. So her love was expressed by feeding him lots of treats.

Here is the story of Minnow's weight-loss walks, told by Sylvia, a pet assistant at the retirement residence where Mae and Minnow live. "When I first met Minnow about two years ago, he weighed close to 19 pounds and did not enjoy going for walks. I started walking him three times a week and slowly increased the distance. He would always walk behind me and was resistant to walking very far. Sometimes he would even try to hide from me when I went to get him to go for his walks. After much encouragement and perseverance, he now weighs 15 pounds and walks with enthusiasm. He loves to go for his walks and proudly trots beside me or even in front of me. Minnow's owner, Mae, is very grateful for his walks and states, 'Walking has helped him so much and keeps him healthy. It has definitely improved his health by giving him much needed exercise. I wouldn't want him to do without his walks.'"

Notes

1. Email exchanges between Phil Zeltzman and Laurie McCauley, May 2010.

2. Ward, E. (2010). *Chow hounds: Why our dogs are getting fatter—A vet's plan to save their lives*. Deerfield Beach, FL: Health Communications.

3. Personal communication between Phil Zeltzman and Lisa Freeman, 2010.

4. DVM Consulting. (2009). FAQ. Balance IT. https://secure.balanceit.com/_clients2/faq.php

8
Start something big!

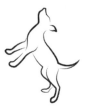

While dog walking can be very rewarding for individuals and their dogs, it can also be fun and beneficial as a group activity. In this chapter, we describe how to create a walking group where both people and dogs can have fun, lose weight, or stay fit. And dogs are the social lubricant that makes it all possible.

Making the commitment

As with any form of exercise, dog walking relies on commitment in order to become part of your life. When you adopt a dog, you commit to giving it a healthy, happy life. Your dog needs exercise. You do too. So in committing to walk your dog, you are also committing to exercise yourself, except that walking your dog won't feel like exercising! Dogs love to walk, so they give you positive feedback along the way. If you commit to walking them, you will benefit in physical, emotional, and social ways. But scientists know that for some people, making a commitment to walking involves more than just having a dog, since many dog owners don't walk their dogs.[1] It is often easier to open the kitchen door to the back yard and let them out to do their business or run around on their own. Many dogs don't walk or run much when they are alone in the back yard. Because they are pack animals, dogs would rather run with another dog or play with their human.

WALKING WITH ALFREDO THE BULLDOG COMES NATURALLY

Walking my eight-year-old American bulldog, Alfredo twice a day with my friends is the only regular exercise I get. While I do avoid processed foods, I never limit my eating in the traditional sense. I never go on a diet.

I find it pretty amazing that by doing something that comes naturally—walking my dog in the fresh air and cooking meals from scratch, I am able to maintain a resting pulse rate in the 50s and I am only about ten pounds away from my ideal weight.

—Sonya, a Pennsylvania resident

Contracts

It may be helpful to make a deal with yourself or others about starting and maintaining a walking program. Writing a contract is simple. It can be a typed document or can even be written on a napkin. The important part is that the contract needs to have goals and be kept in a very visible place. Here is an example:

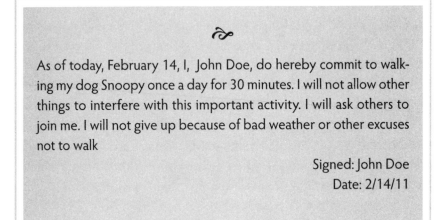

As of today, February 14, I, John Doe, do hereby commit to walking my dog Snoopy once a day for 30 minutes. I will not allow other things to interfere with this important activity. I will ask others to join me. I will not give up because of bad weather or other excuses not to walk

Signed: John Doe
Date: 2/14/11

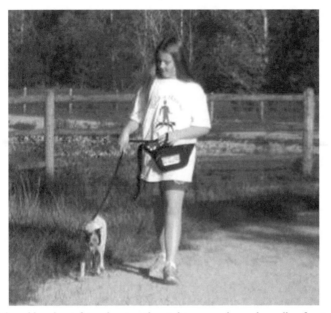

A girl and her best friend enjoy the sights, sounds, and smells of nature.

invite members of these groups to dog walk with you. This can bring an expanded focus to the groups and add a physical activity component that may be lacking. Often such groups revolve around eating. By adding dog walking, you can counteract the effects.

If you are a parent or grandparent, you can start a "walking school bus" in which you walk your children or grandchildren to and from their bus stop or better yet, to and from school. It is natural to add this to your dog walking. Children generally are intrigued by dogs and like the idea of walking with them. Other neighborhood children may want to join. Soon, you could be providing much-needed physical activity for the children while walking the dog. Children who walk to school have been found to be better able to concentrate and listen than children who do not.

Another place where you can start a dog-walking group is at your workplace. Ask your supervisor to support a "bring your dog to work" day each week when workers can in turn bring their dogs and lead their fellow workers in a dog walk during breaks and lunch periods. The "dog of the day" could be provided with a quiet resting place near its owner's work area. Many companies have found that people improve their productivity when there is a dog in the workplace. The dog is a stress reliever and makes the workplace seem friendlier.

Church and other volunteer groups can easily become dog-walking groups to help their members get some exercise. Sponsoring a dog-walking event can be a fundraiser for any group. By charging a small fee and giving participants a free t-shirt and some dog treats, the mission of the group can be supported by people getting physical activity and enjoying their dogs rather than sedentary activities like bingo or fundraising meals.

Dog walking: An effortless change

For most of my life, I have battled fat. Coming from a home where food equaled love, I had to constantly work to keep weight off and keep my bad eating habits in check.

As a professional woman in advertising, I knew the importance of image. I started walking with my dog Fred, but with regular walks, I noticed something magical happening—I wasn't feeling bloated or fat, I was actually feeling healthy and fit. I was also feeling energized, so I decided to walk to work. I began noticing architectural details and landscaped gardens and interesting townhouses.

Walking with Fred made me feel better about myself and the world around me. I met more people and enjoyed the day more. I had more energy. Soon, I was looking forward to my walks with Fred and we became a regular "couple" in our neighborhood.

Fred and I would walk to the park and meet other dog owners and dogs. After a few months of walking, Fred and I were both thinner and healthier. Walking took my mind off food. Dog walking made my life a whole lot healthier and more enjoyable, and it was done without any real effort—it just happened.

—Debra, a Pennsylvania resident

Harness the power of meetup.com

You can use online social networks such as meetup.com to create a weight-loss or dog-walking group or to join an existing group. It's a fascinating tool. Are you interested in meeting other terrier lovers in Chicago? There are three groups. Want to run with your dog in Long Beach, California? Then join Dog-n-Jog every Sunday morning! Would you prefer a dog walking group in New York City? Meetup can provide that, too.

Of course, smaller towns have Meetup groups as well. For example, there is a group of doxie lovers in Allentown, Pennsylvania.

Walking for a cause

Many nonprofit organizations use the concept of walking or running for a cause to raise money or awareness. For example, Erica and Mike and their dog Snoopy, an 18-month-old beagle, walked in an event called Boardwalkin' For Pets in Ocean City, Maryland, for the benefit of the Worchester County Humane Society. The Morris Animal Foundation (www.curecaninecancer.org) sponsors the K9 Cancer Walk in various locations throughout the country to benefit cancer research for dogs. If you are interested in organizing such an event, you can find some resources below.

Fundraising information on the web

- www.fundraising-ideas.org/DIY/dogwalk.htm
- charity.lovetoknow.com/Dog_Walk_Fundraiser
- www.fund-raising-ideas-center.com/dog-fundraising-walkathon. html
- www.relayforlife.org/relay/node/4873
- www.ehow.com/how_4494651_host-dog-walk-fundraiser.html
- www.fundraiserinsight.org/articles/fundraisers-with-dogs.html
- www.runwalkride.com/page.asp?ID=807
- www.fatiguebegone.com/walking_2

Vets as leaders

Veterinarians can also take the lead in starting a walking group. What better way to bond with clients and patients, and have fun with like-minded people? You can meet weekly at a certain time at the vet clinic or at a local park. You can also create special events by connecting with local organizations.

You can all agree, say, once a month, to leave your dogs at home and walk shelter dogs instead. Or you could include members of the local Weight Watchers chapter. Similar ideas are countless. Have fun and be creative!

Members of the vet health care team and their dogs are unfortunately not spared by the overweight epidemic. You could also start a walking group within your own clinic, for example, at lunch time. Even a 15- or 30-minute daily walk will have a positive impact on everybody's weight and the spirit of teamwork at the clinic. And for those fortunate to have a healthy weight, human or canine, it can be a great way to stay fit while supporting your colleagues and bonding with them.

Start something big: Walking loaner dogs

In nearly every town, there is an animal shelter where dogs sit in a cage day in and day out, through no fault of their own. They need exercise and rarely is there enough staff at shelters to provide it. You can volunteer to walk shelter dogs and involve others to do this. It is an incredibly rewarding experience to see a dog leave its cage and spring to life, noticing sights, sounds, and smells as a dog and not as a discarded object. Many cities have programs like the Walk a Hound, Lose a Pound (WAHLAP) dog-walking study, where you can enjoy walking shelter dogs.

In our WAHLAP study, started in 2007, people come to the animal shelter each Saturday morning from April through October to walk the shelter dogs. The program is a partnership between the University of Missouri's College of Veterinary Medicine's Research Center for Human-Animal Interaction (ReCHAI), the Columbia, Missouri Parks and Recreation Department, the Central Missouri Humane Society, and the Missouri Department of Health and Senior Services. A chart below explains the logic model of the program.

The goal of the model is to form a collaboration between the animal shelter, health department, dog rescue groups, pet supply companies, and the parks and recreation department so that they can combine their resources to make the WAHLAP program a highly successful one. These are the Inputs shown in the model. They are the entities that will put resources and time into the program. The next column in the model shows the Activities that are needed to launch a WAHLAP program. The activities are shown across from the Input that can most help with them (e.g., the pet supply companies can provide needed treats to give the dogs during their walks). The next column in the model shows the anticipated short-term outcomes of the program, namely, they show that the program has been well attended, many dogs have received walks, and that there is sufficient equipment and supplies for continued success. The final column in the model describes long-term outcomes. These outcomes reflect the overall values of the program, namely, that dogs get more physical activity, the program results in people who, upon spending time at the shelter for the WAHLAP, decide that they would like to become regular volunteers at the shelter. The program results in more publicity and community awareness of the shelter and needs of shelter dogs, and that the pet supply companies are pleased to be associated with WAHLAP and want a long-term sponsorship. Another desired long-term outcome is that the parks and recreation department values WAHLAP as one of the regular programs that it facilitates each year. Overall, the model shows that when you start with this winning combination of Inputs, and each Input collaborator participates in activities related to its own expertise, WAHLAP can have some wonderful short- and long-term outcomes.

In our Columbia, Missouri Walk a Hound, Lose a Pound program, adults and families preregister to participate through the Parks and Recreation Department's online or telephone registration system. They register for a four-week session and pay a $10.00 fee, which is a donation to the animal shelter. Participants receive a free t-shirt with our program graphic on the front and sponsors' logos on the back. The adults complete a series of questionnaires providing us with research data about themselves, their health, physical activity patterns before and

LOGIC MODEL OF THE WALK A HOUND, LOSE A POUND PROGRAM			
Inputs	**Activities**	**Short-Term Outcomes**	**Long-Term Outcomes**
Animal shelter resources	Identify program Coordinator	Shelter dogs are walked	Increased physical activity in dogs Increased shelter volunteer base Increased adoptions
Public health dept. resources	Get media coverage/market the program	Physically active participants	Participants increase physical activity
Local dog rescue organizations	Help with promotion	Ample participants	Increased visibility of shelter and rescues
Pet supply companies	Obtain supplies	Well-equipped program	Businesses identify with program
Parks & recreation dept. resources	Create or enhance walking trails/ routes	Program attracts participants	Sustainable opportunities for physical activity established

after participating in the program, and dog ownership history. We measure weight and height and check their blood pressure. This research component is something we do as a university research center. You do not need to do this in your program.

We give participants basic instructions on safe leash handling, and provide fanny packs containing dog treats, poop bags, and a card with a number to call in case of emergency. We lead participants through a basic muscle-stretching routine and then match them with a dog compatible with their own physical ability. Shelter dogs participating in the walks are selected by shelter staff based on their adoptability, amicable personality, and ability to be walked. The dog-human teams walk on a nearby shady, crushed-gravel nature trail that we mark with signs designating the quarter-mile, half-mile, three-quarter-mile, and one-mile points. Generally, the walk lasts one hour, although many people come back to get another dog and go for a second or third hour.

People often bring their grandchildren, and community groups focused on children and youth are regular participants. Dog adoptions occur, although people participating in the WAHLAP study are often unable to have dogs due to their life circumstances. What has happened regularly however, is that participants of our study enjoy dog walking so much that they become regular volunteer dog walkers at the animal shelter so that they can walk more frequently than just every Saturday. The project is clearly a win-win situation: people get some exercise and enjoy walking the dogs, and the dogs get valuable socialization with a variety of people and other dogs. The dogs improve their leash-walking skills, making them better candidates as future family members. Shelter staff report that the dogs are calmer and "show" much better to potential adopters the rest of the Saturday—typically the busiest day for adoptions.

WALK A HOUND, LOSE A POUND PARTICIPANT COMMENTS

I want to start running for exercise so this was good for me. It started me exercising and got me started with trainer so I will exercise. I'm telling others about how the program got me exercising.

—A 26-year-old nonexercising woman

I had an epiphany this morning as I was walking from my car to work. It suddenly occurred to me that I was struggling to walk into work. Then I thought back to the Saturday morning walk with the dogs and realized I didn't struggle as much because I was focused on the dogs.

—A 68-year-old woman who walked with loaner dogs

It was a wonderful experience. When I started the program I didn't know what to expect but every week when I don't feel like exercising the pups make me want to walk or run.

—A 36-year-old female owner of five dogs

A word about safety is needed here. While some shelter dogs may have previously mastered their basic obedience skills, many have not. This is important to consider because a good match between the dog's energy level and the walker's physical abilities will help to ensure that walking is a positive experience for both. In particular, shelter dogs may not be adept at loose-lead walking, or heeling, and may pull against the lead, go around the person walking them, or may constantly move from one side of the person to the other. For people with pain or other physical health problems, a dog that is small or less energetic and does not pull against the lead will be the best walking partner for the safety of both. This also applies to people with limitations in balance or an unsteady gait, or to those walking with canes.

Another issue is dog-to-dog aggression. Some shelter dogs may do well in the kennel setting with other dogs, but when out on a lead for a walk, may act out aggressively toward other dogs. It is always advisable to keep the shelter dog away from other dogs and to discourage other people walking dogs to bring their dog over to the shelter dog to "meet and greet." Given that the behavior of the shelter dog is not known, it is better to act conservatively in this situation to prevent problems.

Even if no formal program exists in your community, you can call your local animal shelter and learn how to volunteer to help the dogs get their walks. If you are interested in starting a dog-walking program, you can contact us through our website at www.rechai.missouri.edu to get advice on the steps involved with starting, promoting, and maintaining such a program.

Another loaner opportunity is to volunteer to help someone who cannot walk their own dog. This person may live in your neighborhood and may be elderly or disabled enough not to be able to walk their dog. You can walk their dog for them and feel good about helping yourself, the dog, and its owner. This can add a whole new positive and rewarding dimension to dog walking—the feeling of helping others!

Create a dog-walking business

If you really like dog walking and have an entrepreneurial spirit, you could even start a dog-walking business. Many people are unable to walk their dogs enough. You can be their surrogate dog walker and make some money in the process. Some kick it up a notch and also offer dog-running services, such as Lindsay Stordahl (see her testimonial below).

There are multiple web sites dedicated to the topic, such as www. dogwalker.com (click on Resources and Dog Walking Books). A recent search online for "dog-walking business" generated over 6.5 million links!

A PASSION BECOMES A BUSINESS

I never thought I'd be getting paid to walk and run dogs, but here I am. I can thank my mutt Ace, because once I adopted him I began taking him out on daily six-mile runs. Taking him running was necessary to bond with him, calm him down, and make training more interesting.

During these runs with Ace, I would dream of leaving my office job at the newspaper to hang out with dogs. I realized the problem many pet owners face: how do we find the time to properly exercise our dogs while working so many hours?

It wasn't long before I quit my job and started my own dog-running and -walking business called Run That Mutt. Pursuing my passions for dogs and fitness was one of the best choices I've ever made. I love my job, and at the same time I'm helping dogs lose weight, have fun, and improve their socialization skills.

Hiring a dog walker is a convenient way to provide your dog with some extra fun and exercise. Dogs that are walked every day by their own family members are the happiest and fittest dogs.

When I decided to start a dog-running business, the first dogs I ran were rescue dogs. I've been volunteering to run rescue dogs ever since. Few things are as rewarding as spending time with homeless dogs. They are so grateful for any time I spend with them.

Running has allowed me to be the thinnest, fittest, and healthiest I've ever been. Although I do watch the quantity of sweets and fast food I eat, I also know I can get away with eating whatever I want.

—Lindsay Stordahl, 27, a Fargo, North Dakota resident

To be a good dog walker, you have to be reliable, punctual, self-motivated, and good with dogs and people. You will need excellent people skills to provide superior customer service. You also should be familiar with the area well enough to know where to walk or run safely.

Benefits of such a business are numerous. It's easy to start, with little cost involved. It can be a lot of fun. There are also some significant disadvantages. Come December, it is certainly easier to be a dog walker in California than in Wisconsin. And you can't feel tired and quit after walking a dog for an hour. If you are successful, there will be another dog to walk or run after that, and another one after that. So you need to be athletic enough to sustain the hard work.

As in any business, there will be some paperwork involved. Once your company is created, you will need to figure out the tax consequences and choose a health insurance plan. You will also need liability insurance, which can be obtained through existing associations such as Pet Sitters Associates, LLC (www.petsitllc.com).

For more information about dog exercise and dog training, check out www.RunThatMutt.com and www.ThatMutt.com. To learn more about the business of dog walking, visit www.thatmutt.com/2009/06/08/how-to-start-a-dog-walking-business and www.startadogwalkingbusiness.com.

Notes

1. Johnson, R. A. & Meadows, R. L. (2002). Older Latinos, pets, and health. *Western Journal of Nursing Research, 24*(6), 609-620.

2. Stovitz, S. D., VanWormer, J. J., Center, B. A., & Bremer, K. L. (2005). Pedometers as a means to increase ambulatory activity for patients seen at a family medicine clinic. *Journal of the American Board of Family Practice, 18*, 335-343.

3. Wood, L. & Christian, H. (2011). Dog walking as a catalyst for strengthening the social fabric of the community. In R. A. Johnson, A. M. Beck, & S. McCune (Eds)., *Health benefits of dog-walking* (ch. 4). West Lafayette, IN: Purdue University Press.

9

Create new patterns

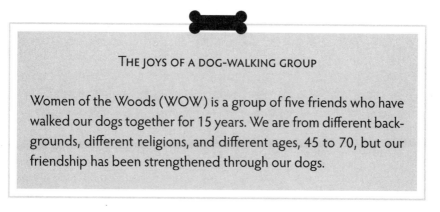

I n this book, we have provided scientific evidence that dog walking can promote health in people and dogs, recommendations for healthy and happy dog walking, and ideas for those who want to implement dog walking on a community level.

Hopefully we have convinced you that by dog walking, you and your dog can reap many benefits. All that is needed to start and maintain a dog-walking activity is a little ingenuity and the desire to do it! By consciously deciding to get off of the sofa, to dog walk, you are making a commitment to your health, your dog's health, or the health of another dog.

Losing weight may actually be easier than keeping it off. Once you have designed new patterns of physical activity and eating, you will create a new lifestyle for yourself and your dog that will help you maintain your desired weight.

THE JOYS OF A DOG-WALKING GROUP

Women of the Woods (WOW) is a group of five friends who have walked our dogs together for 15 years. We are from different backgrounds, different religions, and different ages, 45 to 70, but our friendship has been strengthened through our dogs.

For us, walking has become more than a way to exercise, it has become the way we enjoy our bond, the beauty of nature, the outdoors, and, rather effectively, how we stay in shape. Walking has made us and our dogs stronger, trimmer, and healthier.

I battled overweight my whole life. Growing up in a home where food equaled love meant overeating when I was stressed out and carrying over bad food habits into my adult life. That all changed with dog walking. Now, each and every day, come rain or shine, hail or snow, I start the day with a dog walk.

When we began walking with our first generation of dogs, I was aware of my constant frustration with food and the dieting-overeating routine I often practiced. With walking however, the need to diet had waned. A regular routine of exercise balanced with better eating took me out of a destructive eating cycle and into a world where food was not the enemy—nor was it at center of my universe anymore. It was not an instantaneous transformation, but over time, my food cravings lessened, and I didn't feel the need to eat everything in sight when I was hungry. Actually, I wasn't getting hungry nearly as much as I had in the past. I always believed exercise worked up an appetite, but in reality, just the opposite seemed true. Walking reduced my stress. I wasn't relying on food so much psychologically because food was beginning to take a back seat to another very enjoyable activity: dog walking. I was amazed that something as enjoyable as walking with a dog could be so good for you.

We realized how fit we had become whenever a friend would join us on our walks. They would huff and puff while we walked along almost effortlessly, chatting the entire time. We had stamina, we were in shape, and so were our dogs.

If I missed a walk because of an early meeting, I felt positively sluggish the rest of the day. We all commented on how healthy we felt from walking and how rarely we got sick. I owned my own business and worked 60 or more hours a week, so these walks became a real panacea for me.

Our dogs have benefited from walking as well. Initially, some of our dogs were overweight, but that changed. The bulging tummies were gone and replaced by lean, muscular bodies. Daisy, a yellow Lab, had an operation for hip dysplasia, and the vet commented on what great shape she was in and how her good health contributed to her quick recovery.

Amazingly, all of our dogs died within seven months of each other. We supported each other through each dog's passing and the pain of the loss. Dogs are the best form of preventive medicine, helping us mentally and physically. Now, if I have a stressful day, I grab the leash instead of a candy bar. Walking with my dog has helped balance my life, my body, and my mind and at the same time, has created a bond of friendship that is on its second generation of dogs. We remember our dogs with deep love and thank them for bringing us together and making our lives healthier and happier.

—Debra, a Pennsylvania resident

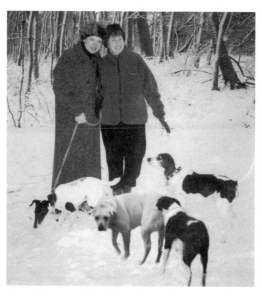

The Women of the Woods celebrate friendship,
good health, and their beloved dogs.

Resources

CHART YOUR HEALTH NUMBERS		
Date	**Current number**	**Target number**
Height		
Weight		
Waist measurement		
BMI		
HDL		
LDL		
Blood pressure		
Steps per day		

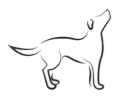

CHART YOUR DOG'S HEALTH NUMBERS		
Date	**Currently**	**Target**
Body weight		
Feel the ribs		
Feel the tail base		
Feel the bony structures		
Belly tuck present?		
Waist present?		
Body Condition Score (specify scale used)		

WEIGHT LOSS TRACKING CHART				
Date	**My weight**	**My weight loss**	**Dog's weight**	**Dog's weight loss**
Ex: May 17	200		35	
Ex: May 30	195	5 lbs	34	1 lb

DAILY DOG WALKING AND ACTIVITY CHART				
Date	**Time**	**Activity and Location**	**Duration/ Number of steps**	**Impressions**
Ex: May 17	*Lunch break*	*Walk in the park*	*30 minutes/ 3000 steps*	*Met John and Fluffy, we all had fun!*

Create a weight loss graph for you and your dog

Weigh yourself and report the number in the top left box below. Then place an X in the box to the right. This is your weight at week 1. The following week, weigh yourself again and report the number below the preceding week, in the left column. Place an X at the intersection of the line with your new weight and the week 2 column. Repeat this process each week. When you join the Xs, you will have a graph showing your weight loss. The same process and chart can be used to track your dog's progress.

WEIGHT LOSS GRAPH										
Weight (lbs)										
Week	1	2	3	4	5	6	7	8	9	10

Determine your ideal weight

It is important to control your body weight as a risk factor. Ideal body weight varies for your gender, height, age, and ethnicity, and beliefs about ideal weight have changed over the years. But the tables below give an estimate.

IDEAL BODY WEIGHT (IN POUNDS)			
MALE		**FEMALE**	
Height	**Ideal Weight**	**Height**	**Ideal Weight**
4' 6"	63 - 77	4' 6"	63 - 77
4' 7"	68 - 84	4' 7"	68 - 83
4' 8"	74 - 90	4' 8"	72 - 88
4' 9"	79 - 97	4' 9"	77 - 94
4' 10"	85 - 103	4' 10"	81 - 99
4' 11"	90 - 110	4' 11"	86 - 105
5' 0"	95 - 117	5' 0"	90 - 110
5' 1"	101 - 123	5' 1"	95 - 116
5' 2"	106 - 130	5' 2"	99 - 121
5' 3"	112 - 136	5' 3"	104 - 127
5' 4"	117 - 143	5' 4"	108 - 132
5' 5"	122 - 150	5' 5"	113 - 138
5' 6"	128 - 156	5' 6"	117 - 143
5' 7"	133 - 163	5' 7"	122 - 149
5' 8"	139 - 169	5' 8"	126 - 154
5' 9"	144 - 176	5' 9"	131 - 160
5' 10"	149 - 183	5' 10"	135 - 165
5' 11"	155 - 189	5' 11"	140 - 171
6' 0"	160 - 196	6' 0"	144 - 176
6' 1"	166 - 202	6' 1"	149 - 182
6' 2"	171 - 209	6' 2"	153 - 187
6' 3"	176 - 216	6' 3"	158 - 193
6' 4"	182 - 222	6' 4"	162 - 198
6' 5"	187 - 229	6' 5"	167 - 204
6' 6"	193 - 235	6' 6"	171 - 209
6' 7"	198 - 242	6' 7"	176 - 215
6' 8"	203 - 249	6' 8"	180 - 220
6' 9"	209 - 255	6' 9"	185 - 226
6' 10"	214 - 262	6' 10"	189 - 231
6' 11"	220 - 268	6' 11"	194 - 237
7' 0"	225 - 275	7' 0"	198 - 242

Source: Rush University Medical Center (www.rush.edu).

WEIGHT OF COMMON DOG BREEDS (IN POUNDS)

Toy dogs

Chihuahua	6
Maltese	4-6
miniature pinscher	10
Pekingese	7-14
Pomeranian	4-6
Yorkshire terrier	7

Small dogs

beagle	26-30
Boston terrier	15-25
Cardigan Welsh corgi	25-38
cocker spaniel	26-34
dachshund	16-32
miniature poodle	11
miniature schnauzer	11-15
Pembroke Welsh corgi	25-30
pug	14-18
Scottish terrier	18-22
shih tzu	9-16
Westie	15-22

Medium dogs

border collie	30-45
Brittany spaniel	30-40
bulldog	40-55
chow chow	40-70
dalmatian	50-59
husky	35-60
Samoyed	37-66
springer spaniel	40-50
standard schnauzer	33-40

Large dogs

Afghan hound	50-60
Bernese mountain dog	90-110
Bouvier des Flandres	60-88
boxer	53-70
Chesapeake Bay retriever	55-80
collie	45-75
Doberman pinscher	64-88
German shepherd	70-95
golden retriever	55-75
greyhound	60-70
Irish setter	60-70
Labrador retriever	55-80
malamute	75-84
standard poodle	44-70
Weimaraner	70-84

Giant dogs

borzoi	55-105
bull mastiff	100-130
Great Dane	120-175
Great Pyrenees	85-100
mastiff	165-198
Newfoundland	100-150
rottweiler	88-110
Saint Bernard	110-200

Based on ranges provided by the American Kennel Club (www.akc.org), individual breed web sites, and information from Hill's Pet Nutrition.

Index

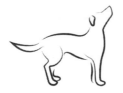